610.733

P9-EEM-196

SH

A Practical Guide to Recruitment and Retention

Skills for Nurse Managers

POINT LOMA NAZARENE UNIVERSITY
WITHDRAWN
RYAN LIBRARY

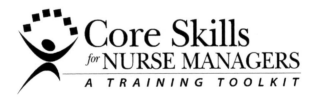

Core Skills *for* NURSE MANAGERS
A TRAINING TOOLKIT

Shelley Cohen, RN, BS, CEN

Dennis Sherrod, EdD, RN

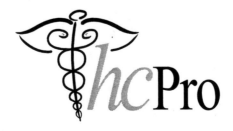

*hc*Pro

A Practical Guide to Recruitment and Retention: Skills for Nurse Managers published by HCPro, Inc.

Copyright 2005 HCPro, Inc.

All rights reserved. Printed in the United States of America.   5   4   3   2   1

1-57839-698-0

No part of this publication may be reproduced, in any form or by any means, without prior written consent of HCPro, Inc., or the Copyright Clearance Center (978/750-8400). Please notify us immediately if you have received an unauthorized copy.

HCPro., Inc, provides information resources for the healthcare industry.

Shelley Cohen, RN, BS, CEN

Dennis Sherrod, EdD, RN

Rebecca Hendren, Associate Editor

Lauren Rubenzahl, Copy Editor

Paul Singer, Layout

Jackie Diehl Singer, Graphic Artist

Jean St. Pierre, Director of Operations

Shane Katz, Cover Designer

Emily Sheahan, Group Publisher

Suzanne Perney, Publisher

Advice given is general. Readers should consult professional counsel for specific legal, ethical, or clinical questions.

Arrangements can be made for quantity discounts. For more information, contact:

HCPro, Inc.

P.O. Box 1168

Marblehead, MA 01945

Telephone: 800/650-6787 or 781/639-1872

Fax: 781/639-2982

E-mail: *customerservice@hcpro.com*

Visit HCPro at its World Wide Web sites:

www.hcpro.com and www.hcmarketplace.com

9/2005
20548

CONTENTS

Contents

Contents

ABOUT THE AUTHORS

Shelley Cohen, RN, BS, CEN

Shelley Cohen, RN, BS, CEN, is the founder and president of Health Resources Unlimited, a Tennessee-based healthcare education and consulting company *(www.hru.net)*. Through her seminars for nursing professionals, Cohen coaches and educates healthcare workers and leaders across the country to provide the very best in patient care. She frequently presents her work on leadership at national conferences.

When she is not speaking or teaching, Cohen works as a staff emergency department nurse and develops educational plans for a local emergency department, including strategies for new graduate orientation. She also writes her monthly electronic publications—*Manager Tip of the Month* and *Triage Tip of the Month*—read by thousands of professionals across the United States.

She is an editorial advisor for *Strategies for Nurse Managers,* published by HCPro, Inc., and is a frequent contributor to *Nursing Management* magazine.

She has a background in emergency, critical care, and occupational medicine. Over the past 30 years, she has worked both as a staff nurse and nurse executive.

When her laptop computer shuts down and her stethoscope comes off, Cohen puts on her child advocacy hat and, with the help of her husband, Dennis, provides foster care to area children.

Dennis Sherrod, EdD, RN

Dennis Sherrod, EdD, RN, serves as the inaugural Forsyth Medical Center Endowed Chair of Recruitment and Retention at Winston-Salem State University in Winston-Salem, NC. He conducts research and program development in the areas of nursing student, faculty, staff, and administration recruitment and retention.

With more than a decade of recruitment and retention experience, he has developed several studies examining young people's perceptions of nursing careers and the ability of newly licensed nurses to make the transition into an evolving healthcare marketplace. He frequently presents his work at conferences across the country, including the National Association of Health Care Recruiters national conferences, *Nursing Spectrum* magazine–sponsored workforce planning events, and *Nursing Management's* National Recruitment and Retention Conference.

Sherrod formerly worked with the NC Center for Nursing, where he served as the director of the North Carolina Institute for Nursing Excellence, the North Carolina Recruitment and Retention Grant Program, and the statewide "Nursing: The Power to Make a Difference" campaign, which encourages youth and minorities to consider nursing and other careers in healthcare.

On the national level, he chaired the Colleagues and Caring Workforce Planning Consortium's recruitment committee and serves on the editorial advisory boards of *Strategies for Nurse Managers* and *Competency Management Advisor,* both published by HCPro, Inc., and the *Nursing Management* journal. On a regional level, he serves on the editorial advisory board of the Southeast edition of *Nursing Spectrum* magazine and the *NC Medical Journal.* He is a member of the American Nurses Association, the Center for American Nurses, the North Carolina Nurses Association, and the North Carolina Association of Healthcare Recruiters.

Sherrod obtained his BS in nursing at Barton College, Wilson, NC, an MSN in nursing education from East Carolina University in Greenville, NC, and an EdD in higher education administration from North Carolina State University in Raleigh, NC.

ACKNOWLEDGMENTS

This book is dedicated to recruiters, managers, nurses and other healthcare providers who commit themselves to making a difference in people's lives each day.

I'd like to acknowledge the steadfast support of Robin, Steven, and Devon that allows me to soar, and the daily discussions with Pete that keep me well-grounded.–Dennis Sherrod

Many thanks to all of the managers I meet in person and via e-mail who are so willing to share their challenges. These same nurse leaders have the courage to listen to staff perspectives and are eager to meet their needs to improve retention and recruitment. The changing viewpoint of placing the new graduate nurse in specialty areas remains a challenge for many staff nurses to embrace. These same leaders have stood strong in the concept of "growing your own" and are to be commended for supporting our future nurses.

I would like to particularly thank Laurie Maxwell, Director of Emergency Services at NorthCrest Medical Center, for demonstrating the important role the nurse leader plays in the world of nursing retention and recruitment.

Behind every writer is a very patient and supportive person who gives us the space and time we need to produce our work. My husband, Dennis, is always there offering support and encouragement in all my professional and personal endeavors. His unconditional love is a strong reminder of the power we have when we are not just the caregiver, but also when we are truly cared for.–Shelley Cohen

Chapter 1

THE REVOLVING DOOR: THE DISADVANTAGE OF HIGH STAFF TURNOVER

Learning objective

After reading this chapter, the participant should be able to

- identify the major disadvantages of high staff turnover

Case study: Staff in, staff out

As I was driving home from work one night, all I could think about was how to find people to fill the empty slots for the night shift. With my best clinical resource person leaving in two weeks, night shifts were going to be pretty naked as far as skills go. I tried to concentrate on the drive, but my mind kept reverting back to the nurses I had lost in the past year. For each one, I kept asking myself, "What could I have done differently? Did they leave because of me, the organization, or their coworkers? What was going on that was pushing my nurses out the door?" I dreaded the thought of the time I would have to spend going through applications and interviews and all the stresses that go along with that process.

I promised myself that this time things would be different; this time, I would not wait for people to tell me they wanted to leave. Instead, I would find a way to identify what I could do to keep them. For those who are still on staff with me, I would create a process I could use to work with them to ensure that they don't become a new statistic in the revolving door of staff.

Make the change—you can stop the door from revolving

How many times have you promised yourself that next time you would handle things differently? Yet when that time approaches, we revert back to our old and comfortable behaviors.

Now is the time for you to commit to changing your recruitment and retention attitude and behavior. At a time when the facility down the street may simply dangle more money per hour to recruit staff, you need ammunition you can dangle back to keep staff from moving out the door. Therefore, recruitment and retention needs your ongoing attention.

The disadvantages of high turnover

For every nurse you keep, consider the savings in time and money that did not have to go toward hiring and orienting a replacement nurse. Also consider that lower turnover places less stress on the existing staff. As managers, we know all too well that staff already feel overwhelmed by their daily responsibilities. For most of them, orienting a new nurse feels like a burden rather than a privilege. Even once the orientation process is underway, someone still has to fill in for the nurse who left, you may find yourself begging staff to pick up more hours, and your budget changes as you pay overtime for coverage on top of the salary of the new person being oriented.

New managers have not been given the education, tools, and resources to manage recruitment and retention. Many organizations now realize the important role you play, not only in retention, but also the likelihood that your staff will recommend their place of employment to others. This book will provide you with resources and will guide you in using leadership skills to embrace the concept that you are the number one recruiting officer for the organization.

Changing perceptions

The first step is to be realistic. You may need to change your attitudes and perceptions regarding keeping and recruiting talented staff. If any of the following thoughts are still in the back of your mind, make an attitude adjustment before you can hope to find success with your recruitment and retention strategies:

- "What more do they want from me? They're getting paid for what they do."
- "In my day, we were just grateful to get the job we wanted."

- "I'm getting really tired of 'making nice' just to keep people from leaving."
- "This new generation expects so much from us, but they are the first to say no to working a weekend or holiday shift."

These are the realities of nursing practice today. We are in the midst of a national nursing shortage, even if some areas of the country are experiencing more challenges than others. Our work force is getting older, and the new, young entries are from a generation that knows how to negotiate to get what they want from an employer. The role of the nurse manager has changed—you are more of a leader now than ever before.

Nurse managers play a key role

Realize the importance of your leadership role. You can find a way to ensure that the revolving door only moves when you want it to. You can embrace the research and evidence about work environments and how they directly affect staff's perceptions. If money were the only thing people wanted, then why do so many nurses report being dissatisfied with where they work, the resources available, and the managers to whom they report?

One of the most commonly uttered phrases in the nursing tradition is, "that's how we've always done it," but it is time to go ahead and break your traditions. It is time to embrace new processes that will reap benefits not only for nurses, but also for patient care. You are taking a giant step forward as you embrace the contents of this book.

"Recruitment without retention is a colossal waste of time, effort, energy, money, and good nurses."
—Rita. H Losee, ScD, Med, RN[1]

References

1. Rita. H. Losee, ScD, Med, RN, "Viewpoint," *American Journal of Nursing* 104, no. 5, (May 2005): 13.

Chapter 2

Embracing Diversity in the Workplace

Learning objectives

After reading this chapter, the participant should be able to
- identify characteristics of a diverse workforce
- discuss strategies for managing diversity in your organization

Identifying your diverse work force

Franklin Thomas, former president and CEO of the Ford Foundation, wrote, "One day our descendants will think it incredible that we paid so much attention to things like the amount of melanin in our skin, or the shape of our eyes, or our gender instead of the unique identities of each of us as complex human beings."[1]

The differences in your staff make all the difference in the world. The communities we serve are becoming more diverse, and the goal of most employers is to provide a work force that reflects the people, families, and groups that make up your client base.

When people think of diversity, we often think of the differences that are visually apparent, such as age, gender, ethnicity, and physical disability. But diversity also includes differences in religion, nationality, citizenship, socio-economic status, educational background, sexual orientation, and political affiliation. Work experiences, abilities, skills, competencies, values, personalities, preferences, and dislikes are different in each individual as well. All these dimensions and more combine to form the unique identities of each member of your staff.

Diversity is not skin-deep

There are even more variations to be found within these differences. Consider the educational background of your nursing staff—registered nurses have three distinct entry points: diploma, associate, and baccalaureate programs. Nationality is another interesting dimension. There may be values and customs you share with colleagues from the United States, but you also differ depending on whether your peers grew up in a rural or urban area, or whether they have worked in the north, south, east, or west of the country or in a United States territory.

The diversity that each healthcare professional brings to the workplace is a result of the individual's life-long cultural, educational, and work experiences. You will see differences in lifestyle, preferences, thinking, and decision-making. Each member of your staff will process information in different ways and at different speeds. The challenge for you is to provide a forum to encourage expression of different opinions and ideas.

Embracing the diversity of your staff involves recognizing and appreciating personal dimensions and interpersonal dynamics. Cultural beliefs, traditions, and practices combine to form unique social identities for each one of us. A commitment to valuing diversity also requires that we address continuing disparities in healthcare, racism, and sexism and that we provide equal opportunity for all. Valuing and accepting the individual differences of the people who work on a unit provide a wide and ample array of options to address evolving healthcare challenges in increasingly diverse communities.

Building a case for diversity

A diverse healthcare work force offers many benefits. Having a variety of viewpoints and perspectives among your staff allows for more creative ideas and solutions—two heads are better than one only when one is not a duplicate of the other.

Indeed, you should long for staff with a variety of backgrounds and experiences and who express different thoughts and ideas. You may achieve faster decisions if everyone suggests the same idea, but differences of opinion and discussion produce better problem-solving options. Additionally, having staff that reflect the culture and life experiences of the patients you serve will help you identify the specific needs and interests of your patient population. It also can increase profitability by attracting those different patient groups. Many people prefer to have a practitioner with whom they can identify deliver their healthcare. Thus, having diverse staff with extensive knowledge of diverse patients can help you individualize your care to meet the needs of different groups. Knowledge and understanding of specific groups also helps to improve your quality of patient care.

Employees benefit from a diverse work environment as well. They can be challenged to explore a wider range of social, cultural, emotional, intellectual, spiritual, and economic perspectives. When respect for individual differences is promoted in this way, staff members develop a fuller appreciation of a changing society and adapt better to those changes. Employees exposed to a colleague's complex differences are better prepared to address evolving changes in increasingly diverse communities and global economies.

Learning about other cultural beliefs and practices allows us to expand our own cultural experiences. Understanding and appreciating others' cultural beliefs can decrease interpersonal conflict and improve teamwork. Diversity makes great business sense in healthcare settings, especially when leadership and economic opportunity is equally available to talented and qualified individuals from all backgrounds.

Demonstrating the value of diversity

Include in your employee orientation a session that helps new employees understand that each person has complex, multiple identities that can influence patterns of socialization and affiliation. Ask new employees what attracted them to you as an employer. Review your mission and vision statements to make sure they clearly state your organizational value for inclusiveness, pluralism, and diversity for employees and the community you serve. Help your staff understand that your unit work culture supports acceptance and appreciation, equal treatment and opportunity, individual contributions, personal growth, respect, and trust.

Ways to increase diversity

Verbalize in staff meetings and public forums the benefits of differences and similarities within your organization and community. Develop relationships with institutions that have diverse membership. If you have identified a specific need to recruit African-American nursing students, develop a partnership with a historically black college or university. You also may want to establish partnerships with health profession programs across the country that target

Latino students. Include schools and organizations with diverse membership as integral recruitment sources.

Establish local chapters of professional association groups who target minority nurses and encourage staff to participate. These associations include the American Assembly of Men in Nursing, National Association of Hispanic Nurses, National Black Nurses Association, or Philippine Nurses Association of America. Develop mentoring programs with organizational staff and community leaders.

Practice what you preach

If you value something, you must act upon it. That is to say, an organization that truly values diversity cannot define diversity as a value and then do nothing about it. Instead, such organizations must provide equal treatment and access to resources and decision-making regardless of race, ethnicity, sexual orientation, and physical disability. You also must develop policies that allow staff, managers, and administrators to address racism, sexism, homophobia, and other forms of oppression.

Consider developing and implementing strategies that publicly recognize cultural traditions of different groups within your organization. For example, you can establish a specific number of paid holidays but allow flexibility in when your staff choose to take them. Not all of your employees will celebrate Thanksgiving or Christmas, and they may prefer to take those holidays at a different time. What a great advantage of diversity—you have staff willing to work Thanksgiving and Christmas!

Listen and learn

Seek to understand how groups relate to issues of power, privilege, and oppression. Remember that each of us looks at issues from our own cultural references. It's entirely fine to ask an employee to "Tell me how you feel about…" or "I'd like to learn more about… " Additionally, if an individual brings up issues relating to power, privilege, oppression, or unfair treatment, ask them to describe a specific scenario so you can determine a method of corrective action.

Watch for nonverbal cues from people. If you make a statement you feel is not offensive but verbal cues tell you that it might have been perceived in a negative manner, then acknowledge that your comment appears to have been received in a way you did not mean. Seek a deeper understanding of how your statement or behavior might be perceived by other groups or cultures.

Establishing common ground

Develop and support processes that allow employee groups to address priorities specific to the group, and at the same time help them to find common ground with organizational goals, concerns, and issues. Therefore, identify groups in your organization, and hold open forum meetings to determine issues and improvements. Ask questions such as the following:

- What can be done to improve your satisfaction?
- What limits your productivity here?
- How can we improve your creativity?
- Can you describe examples of unfair treatment you have experienced here?
- What types of power, privilege, or oppression issues have you observed here?

Do not send personal invitations based on your guess of which groups your employees might be affiliated with; instead, post notices for a 'None of us is strong as all of us'–type forum series, with a different group focus each meeting. Encourage employees to attend and provide input. Have someone there to document the issues, and upon conclusion of the series, provide follow-up and acknowledgement of changes and improvements.

Demonstrating commitment to diversity

A first impression is made in less than three seconds. When potential employees are making decisions concerning employment, they review your organization based on their own cultural backgrounds, perceptions, and preferences. And although they don't have to see someone who looks exactly like them, they do want to see an individual or group with whom they can readily identify. If you're targeting specific groups, make sure your recruitment personnel can identify easily with the target groups. This strategy is not restricted to race and ethnic background, so invite a seasoned nurse who is an alumnus of a specific nursing program to attend the recruitment event. Or, if you're highlighting your orientation or residency program, include a recent successful graduate who readily identifies with students about to graduate.

Increasing diversity among nursing leadership

Interested candidates look for diversity throughout your organization's work force, including among your leadership at the manager, administrator, and board of director levels. However, diversity among nursing leadership continues to be a challenge in most hospitals and healthcare facilities. Consider a fast-track program to increase leadership diversity by identifying nurses early on in their careers who demonstrate promising leadership potential. Coach, groom, and develop their leadership competencies and skills to move them quickly into leadership roles in your organization.

Increase representation

When recruiting diverse groups in media campaigns, consider the types of media that target the groups you seek. Remember, we choose our interactions based upon our cultural backgrounds. If you are attempting to reach ethnic groups, consider publications and cultural events that target those groups. If you're interested in reaching older prospective candidates, you might consider advertising in a publication of the AARP.

Review all organizational media and advertising to make sure employee diversity is demonstrated. For example, don't distribute a nurse recruitment video that depicts only African-American nursing assistants and Caucasian registered nurses and nurse managers. Rather, show that all groups have growth potential in your organization and that there are no career ceilings for any individual or group.

Highlight your organization's commitment to diversity

Make a conscious effort to demonstrate the full range of your organizational diversity in all of your public relations strategies.

My organization values diversity because we do the following:

✓ Make a special effort to recruit individuals from ethnic backgrounds
✓ Advertise in local ethnic newspapers or newsletters
✓ Advertise in ethnic magazines or journals
✓ Offer cultural events in our facility
✓ Encourage staff to attend community cultural events
✓ Sponsor community cultural events
✓ Have formal partnerships with ethnic-focused professional associations or organizations

---

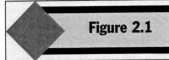

Figure 2.1 — **U.S. registered nurse ethnicity and gender**

Registered nurses	Population
Ethnicity:	
• White: 86.6% • Black: 4.9% • Hispanic: 2.0% • Asian/Pacific Islander: 3.7% • American Indian/Alaskan Native: 0.5% • Two or more races: 1.2%	• White: 75.1% • Black: 12.3% • Hispanic: 12.5% • Asian/Pacific Islander: 3.7% • American Indian/Alaskan Native: 0.9% • Two or more races: 2.4%
Gender:	
• Female: 94.6% • Male: 5.4%	• Female: 49.1% • Male: 50.9%
National Sample Survey of Registered Nurses, March 2000[2]	U.S. Census Data, 2000[3]

The untapped recruitment potential of diversity

Breakdown of nursing demographics

Nursing has historically been, and continues to be, a female-dominated profession. Upon analysis of ethnic and gender proportions of the registered nurse work force, it is immediately apparent that the ethnic and gender makeup of nursing does not reflect the general population. The data contained in Figure 2.1 show that the nursing work force is 86.6% white, compared to 75.1% for the population as a whole. Nurses are also 94.1% female, compared to 49.1% of the general population.

A look at the data shows that there is significant recruitment potential among non-white and non-female populations. Although multiple and complex issues affect nurse recruitment trends on the national level, to remain competitive, you must ensure that your work place culture is appealing and attractive to a diverse nurse workforce.

Our unit's diversity principles

- Employees are hired based upon skills and competencies required for desired organizational outcomes
- Staff are managed in a fair and equitable manner, regardless of age, gender, ethnicity, race, physical disabilities, religion, nationality, socio-economic status, educational background, sexual orientation, and political affiliation
- Unit culture promotes individual expression of thought
- Unit manager provides a variety of speakers and community partners

---

Managing diverse work forces

"If we are to achieve a richer culture, rich in contrasting values, we must recognize the whole gamut of human potentialities, and so weave a less arbitrary social fabric, one in which each diverse human gift will find a fitting place."[4]

As a manager of diversity, create an environment that values and uses talents, skills, and contributions of people with different backgrounds, experiences, and perspectives. Identify diversity as a core component of organizational leadership and leadership development. Include criteria related to diversity on performance evaluations, such as "demonstrates ability to work with a variety of colleagues" or "demonstrates value for different thoughts, ideas, and preferences."

Also incorporate principles of diversity into staff meetings. As you discuss the importance of recognizing differences in clients, affirm the importance of recognizing and appreciating differences and similarities among peers and colleagues. Help staff understand how diverse thoughts and ideas are a perfect fit with quality improvement models. Always look for ways to improve quality and efficiency—and note that a variety of ideas helps to provide solutions to everyday challenges and problems.

Educate

Managers must ensure that knowledge of cultural diversity is available to all levels of staff through continuing education, discussion groups, and other educational strategies. Observe for signs of bias and assumptions. When you hear statements such as, "That doesn't affect me. We don't have much diversity here," or "I'm not prejudiced, but they just don't fit in," be prepared to talk about the importance of diversity.

Also watch for signs of ethnocentrism, stereotyping, or prejudice in conversations, attitudes, and actions. Stereotypes are distorted thoughts or views toward members of a group or people. Ethnocentrism is a belief that one's group or culture is superior to others. Prejudice is an attitude or belief about a person or group based upon stereotypes. Equip your staff to identify and address these misperceptions on a daily basis.

Assess individual bias and assumptions, and develop rules of engagement in your staff meetings. Ask questions about different cultures and preferences. Be aware that each culture or group may have values, beliefs, customs and traditions, behaviors, and words and language that are important to them. Determine how your staff's cultures and backgrounds influence the way they deliver patient care. Listen to employees and provide opportunities for them to offer their thoughts. Be careful not to assume that no response or silence signifies understanding or agreement.

Ensure that difference doesn't lead to exclusion

Consider what can happen in work situations, particularly when a new member who is considered to be "different" enters the group. Staff may exclude those identified as "different" by not acknowledging them, speaking to them, or including them in unit activities. Staff also may deny that differences exist. They may encourage individuals to suppress their differences or to assimilate or conform to majority standards. If you hear an employee say, "If they want to live in America, they should act like Americans," engage that employee in the question of what exactly an American acts like. This chapter has already established that Americans have many dimensions.

Don't ask, don't tell

Many employment settings tolerate differences through a superficial "live and let live" atmosphere. This is similar to the "Don't ask, don't tell" policy used by the armed forces. This type of situation will only promote superficial interaction among your staff and can hide simmering problems.

Mutual adaptation

The most effective option is mutual adaptation, where every employee accommodates change. This option is based on the idea that cultural identities should be maintained and valued rather than discarded or ignored. Engaging employees in dialogue about differences helps to build trusting, productive relationships among your staff.

Most small children are taught to treat others as they themselves would want to be treated. But as adults, we discover that not everyone wants to be treated as we prefer to be treated. Instead, we must learn to treat others the way *they* prefer to be treated. Therefore, ask questions and listen to the response—your staff will be delighted to share their preferences.

Respectful and committed employees

Realize that people are both the same and different, and each of us lives, practices, leads, and is influenced by cultures established by others. Although you want to create a culture that recognizes individual differences, you also want each of your staff to be fully engaged in and committed to a common goal of providing quality patient care.

Embracing diversity requires the consistent and diligent integration of diversity strategies into your workplace setting. These strategies must include all employees and be supported by nurse managers and administration. The goal is to recruit and retain staff based upon their merits and contributions to quality patient care. You must not focus on a specific number of individuals from one group or another but rather on individuals who have the skills to help accomplish your desired outcome of excellent patient care.

References

1. Gloria Steinem, *"Outrageous Acts and Everyday Rebellions,"* (New York: Henry Holt and Company, 1983): 393.

2. U.S. Department of Health and Human Services, National Sample Survey of Registered Nurses, *http://bhpr.hrsa.gov/nursing/sampsurvpre.htm.*

3. U.S. Census Bureau, *US Census Data, www.census.gov/,* March 2000.

4. Margaret Mead, *Sex and Temperament in Three Primitive Societies* (New York: HarperCollins: 1935).

Chapter 3

DEVELOPING NURSE MANAGERS AND LEADERS

Learning objectives

After reading this chapter, the participant should be able to

- identify strategies to support and develop nurse managers
- recognize warning signs that a new nurse manager is in need of support, guidance, and direction
- implement strategies that managers can use to show staff that you make time for them

How administration can support and retain the nurse manager

Organizations devote much time and effort to retention at the staff level, but they have forgotten the importance of retaining the middle manager. We have neglected to give adequate attention, nurturing, and support to the very people we hope will retain the nurses we recruit. An organization's recruitment and retention goals need to include the leaders who oversee the nursing staff.

Nurse managers' challenges

An administrator may view nurse managers as leaders who should not need handholding to want to stay in their jobs, but it is important for them to put themselves in the shoes of today's nurse manager. In many facilities, nurse managers face daily struggles to manage their workloads and support their limited staff. We must make it a priority to support this vital group of employees and meet their professional and personal desires.

Promotion without training

Part of the challenge is that many nurse managers and leaders are selected for their positions based on their clinical skills, rather than on their leadership capabilities. We cannot expect people to stay and excel in positions for which they have no skills or training.

On the other end of the spectrum are those managers with appropriate leadership experience who accept positions. You are relieved to finally fill open positions, so return to focus on your own job responsibilities. The new managers have the qualifications for the roles, have performed them well elsewhere, and will, you hope, ask for help or support if they need it.

Such misperceptions can result in new managers who are unhappy because they sense a lack of administrative support. Imagine being a newly hired manager in a facility where you do not yet have a feel for processes, the systems, or the team. Your new staff will test you to see how you measure up, the medical staff may not cooperate, and you'd like to fit in with your peer group, but no formal introductions were made through your administrative leader, so now you feel isolated and unprepared. Would you want to hang around through the 90 day probationary period?

Establish goals and expectations

Leadership development plays a vital role in the success and satisfaction of nurse leaders, and will directly affect the retention of all, not just the newly hired. Although retention efforts should focus on both new and seasoned managers, how you approach your retention efforts will at times be directed by their length of employment within the organization.

Tips for developing nurse leaders

- Have senior administration allot specific time for retention efforts related to mid-level managers.

- Engage managers in discussion to gain input on their individual requirements as they relate to professional development and personal needs.

- Identify the particular skills that managers need to enhance their productivity and improve patient outcomes on their units. Provide the resources for them to attain these skills.

- Clarify and define success in their role from both your perspective and theirs.

- Schedule ongoing formal and informal communication opportunities between the nurse manager and the person to whom they report.

Case study: Sink or swim

James was hired two years ago as the nurse manager for a 28-bed medical-surgical floor. He had four years of similar management experience at a facility in another state. Because of his previous experience, James was simply put through the hospital orientation program and then was off and running. As his administrator, you find yourself not only frustrated with complaints about him, but also disappointed in his inability to make things happen.

You schedule a meeting with James to share your concerns and to determine whether it is best for him to continue in this role. At the meeting you discover that James is not only unhappy with his position, but that he has put out feelers for openings at another facility. You ask him why he didn't come to you about this sooner and whether there is anything in particular that is making him feel the need to leave.

Realize that both you and James perceive his role from two completely different perspectives. You may wonder why he is unable to attend the nurse management team meetings on a monthly basis, yet without your knowledge, he may have been assigned to a committee that had conflicting dates, and James may have felt that he should try to attend some meetings from both committees. He may have been uncomfortable discussing it with you for fear that you would perceive that he couldn't handle it. Without regular ongoing communication, both of you will continue to have misperceptions about what to expect.

Orienting the new manager

Regardless of where you are in a work relationship with the managers who report to you, there are important points to consider:

Accurate job description: Is there a job description in writing that clarifies expectations? The job description may have been written several years ago and may not reflect the current issues that require oversight of the manager. Review the job description with the manager annually

Identify management and leadership skills: Develop a process to identify a new manager's basic knowledge of management and leadership skills. Include terminology related to fiscal issues and formulas to calculate staffing and budget needs. This assessment will provide a work frame in which to develop goals and identify the supportive and educational needs of the manager. [See figure 3.1 for a sample assessment tool to measure new managers' knowledge/skills.]

Establish goals: Set goals to help managers see their accomplishments and allow you to feel their progress as leaders. It also allows them to feel they are accomplishing something. [See figure 3.2 for suggested goals.]

Provide support from peers: Assign all new managers a mentor from their peer group. Consider having a hotline that managers can access and with which they can leave a message if they need resources or advice on an employee issue. The last thing you want is managers spending time trying to resolve something on which another manager can immediately direct them. The following scenarios would be well served by a hotline:

- *I can't get Information Systems to print me off my monthly budget report—they keep telling me managers don't get a copy.*

- *I need to refer an employee to the EAP program, and I can't get the counselor to return my phone calls.*

- *To whom can I refer a staff member who is interested in going to nursing school and is looking for some scholarship resources?*

Equip them with tools: Provide them with the tools and resources they need to be successful in their roles. Provide a resource/reference library with books that enhance leadership skills.

Offer support and perspective: Schedule regular one-on-one meetings. Make sure you have reviewed the reasons for which previous managers have left, even if you disagreed with their perceptions of the situation. They may offer valuable insight into how you can support the new manager.

| Figure 3.1 | **New manager foundation knowledge/skills assessment** |

Please rate your level of comfort in independently performing the following functions/tasks:
1 = No experience with this
2 = Have a little experience, but I will need guidance
3 = I have some experience, but I will need a resource to go to the first few times
4 = I feel very comfortable with this, but I prefer that you check it the first time
5 = I can independently perform this

1. JCAHO regulations
1 2 3 4 5

Knowledge of those that apply to the clinical areas for which you are responsible
Ability to interpret standards
Knowledge of resources available to assist with implementation of new standards

2. Performance improvement
1 2 3 4 5

Ability to identify indicators for improvement processes
Ability to determine which processes require improvement
Knowledge of techniques to involve staff in the improvement process
Knowledge of relating performance improvement to JCAHO requirements

3. Fiscal responsibilities
1 2 3 4 5

Understand budgeting terms and processes
Ability to relate month-to-date numbers to year-to-date figures
Capable of calculating FTE's and other data related to fiscal concerns

4. Computer skills
1 2 3 4 5

Ability to use Excel spreadsheets and Word documents
Ability to maintain files, flow sheets, and charts regarding staff and quality review
Knowledge of resources available through the Internet

5. Human resources
1 2 3 4 5
Feel comfortable managing conflict on the unit
Understand regulatory rules regarding termination and hiring
Ability to interview effectively

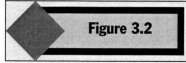

Figure 3.2	30-day goals

Goals for new manager: Sandra. Re-review with Sandra at meeting on November 16.

1. Learn payroll system and independently do employee payroll for pay period ending November 15
2. Meet with CFO to review budget process for your department
3. Meet with medical director of your unit to initiate collaborative efforts regarding patient outcomes

Creating goals for all managers helps them stay focused and feel that they are accomplishing things that matter.

Providing support, guidance, and direction

When you explore retention issues for staff at this level of responsibility, the administrative team must make time to ask the managers some key questions. This simple action sends a message that the manager's input is important and that his or her role is valued by the overall organization. Have them ask the following questions:

- What is the one thing this organization provides you that has the greatest impact on maintaining your employment here?

- When you talk with others about how satisfied you are with your job, what are the things we do that give you that feeling of satisfaction?

- What do you think are some of the reasons other managers have left?

- If you had the power to add one benefit, process, or system related to your position, what would it be?

We generally consider leadership development to be simply providing education, resources, and tools for the manager, but it also includes picking up clues about whether managers are so overwhelmed that they cannot function in their roles. For retention efforts to be successful, there has to be a place for helping managers who feel they are in over their head. Be alert to some of the warning signs that a manager needs to be thrown a life preserver.

Warning signs of stress may include

- appearing unhappy or tired, losing or gaining weight, and being unable to focus or take direction
- being constantly unable to meet deadlines
- frequently canceling meetings set up with own manager
- exhibiting negative non-verbal behavior
- own staff going to other managers or the administrative team with concerns

---

Don't assume that things will be better next week. Make the effort now to confront your concerns and get help and support for the manager. You may do so through your employee assistance program, some time off, or a combination of administrative support and setting new, more realistic expectations.

Professional development—ensuring return on your investment

Some of the efforts organizations make to retain or recruit the mid-level nurse manager are unsuccessful. To better understand why, review typical scenarios that reflect some of the challenges and obstacles getting in the way of your efforts.

Case study: High hopes v. everyday reality

You have invested registration fees, airline and hotel costs, and paid time away for Sandra to attend a national meeting for nurse managers. She returned enthusiastic, rejuvenated, and full of ideas and new networking resources. Her outlook quickly changed, however, when reality set in—she returned to find her desk buried under piles of mail, her inbox full of requests from staff, and the phone's ever-flashing red light.

Such situations suck the enthusiasm out of a mid-level manager. Therefore, instead of approaching the issue that way, take the opportunity to help develop Sandra's organizational skills prior to her attending the meeting. Share some helpful tips that you use in your daily practice to manage paper flow, phone calls, and other office tasks when you are away so that the conference remains a boon instead of becoming another headache.

For example, you can hold a quick, informal meeting in which you help Sandra discuss her expectations of her workload upon her return and prepare ways to manage it. Offer ways for her to remotely pick up e-mail and phone calls at the end of each conference day. Also suggest that

- she delegate a senior staff member who will follow up on priority concerns she identifies from e-mail and phone calls

- she work with another manager from her peer group so each can cover for the other when away for periods of time

- she post her schedule for staff prior to departure

- she schedules a catch-up day when she returns to work

Also note that the knowledge Sandra obtained at a conference will be valuable to other managers, so have her share her experiences at a managers' meeting. Schedule a specific date for this presentation, and if the conference sells audiotapes, have Sandra bring the one that reflects what she feels was the most pertinent information of the conference. Using such a medium encourages other managers to participate in ongoing professional development. Another benefit of sending Sandra to the conference is that doing so sends her a message that her role is important—that the organization is willing to invest in her ongoing education and professional development.

Mentor the manager

Another way to support managers is to assign them a preceptor or mentor. Typically, the mentor or preceptor should come from within the manager's peer group and can be effective and supportive if administration considers the following:

- Preceptor selection should not be based on tenure with the organization, rather, it should be based on skills, character, and support for the mission.

- Administrative managers should work with preceptors to develop a written assessment tool to identify baseline knowledge of both newly hired and established managers.

- Administrative managers should never assume that all is going well with the preceptor simply because you have not heard otherwise. Body language reveals things that managers may be uncomfortable about discussing proactively, so meet with them regularly, in person, to hear their perception of how things are going.

Case study: Ineffective mentor

Juanita has been a nurse manager at the facility for more than 15 years. She is well liked by her staff, the medical staff respect her, and administration can always count on her for help with last-minute issues. She has been assigned as a preceptor to Hank, who was hired as a nurse manager four months ago. After seeing them work together and collaborate at meetings, you walk away feeling good about the match. You meet with Hank monthly to discuss issues related to his department, and it appears that he is easily becoming a part of the organization. He also has shared with you that his family is well settled into the community and that his wife is working locally.

Look below the surface

Is there a problem? If you don't ask, you will never know. It's worth being cautious about how new managers are doing, as they may not want to share with you what is really happening.

For example, if you provide Hank with an evaluation tool that he can use to review his preceptor, he may not want to reflect any negative comments on a peer, especially in writing. Therefore, to find out how he is really doing, schedule a meeting in which the two of you can discuss openly the realities of his new position.

Juanita may be doing a fine job of offering support to Hank and teaching him, for example, how to process payroll and perform other such tasks. However, because she has held the position for so long and because this facility is the only place where she has been a manager, she has always done things a certain way, and it is a challenge for her to be aware of options. These facts mean that when Hank wants to discuss new protocols, standards, or approaches to staff issues, he gets a common response from Juanita: "That is not how we do things around here."

Precepting is not a one-way learning process—Juanita could learn something from Hank as well. Consider using some of the prompters on the manager follow-up sheet (see Figure

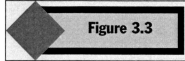

Figure 3.3 — Manager follow-up prompters

The following questions can be used for new and seasoned nursing management staff:

- Now that you have been here for a few months, do you feel that having _____ as a preceptor has been helpful?
- Because we each have our own personal style of managing, do you feel you can be yourself freely at this point? What have you implemented/done in your area(s) that you realize other managers here are not doing?
- What has been the most surprising thing to you about this organization?
- What skills are you interested in learning that we can help you with by providing the resources for you to obtain them?
- Because I work with so many different managers, it is a challenge at times to know specifically what each of you need from me as far as time and other support. What can I do or provide for you that will help you in your job?
- Can you think of something we have expected of you as part of your job that was an unrealistic expectation?

3.3) to help you get to the pertinent information when you have this discussion with a new manager.

Successful leadership development requires continual effort

Leadership development is not a one-stop process. For it to be successful, it must be ongoing, and there must be commitment to it from the top. Your commitment becomes evident through your actions, not through what you may say you will do. Therefore, have a process to ensure that you follow through on requests, issues, and other staff concerns. Doing so is vital to the perceptions of managers who feel that their employer cares about them and cares about what they need.

Improving interview skills

Although selecting new staff to add to the team is one of the most important roles nurse managers play in relation to recruitment and retention, their interview skills typically are not addressed. Nurse managers often are assumed to have such skills when they do not.

Therefore, an important part of developing nurse managers is to help them acquire the skills to choose appropriate staff.

For example, although nurse managers are under intense pressure to fill vacant positions, we need to move away from hiring people because their licenses are clean and they can start right away. The pressure to fill slots can never be an excuse to hire any person who appears qualified. Support managers in making decisions that benefit the entire facility when they choose not to hire particular individuals—the long-term effects on morale and patient safety are not worth the trial-and-error option of hiring individuals who are not right for the job or the situation.

Practical tips to improve hiring skills

Use leadership development to improve the interview and hiring process by educating managers and providing them with resources and tools to guide them through the interview process. Do the following:

- Incorporate interview scenarios in your monthly management meetings

- Ask each manager to bring to the meeting what they feel is the most effective question they ask at an interview

- Provide reference materials that can help the manager improve interview techniques and approaches

- Demonstrate the importance of hiring for character versus hiring for skill through your own interview techniques

- Work with all your nurse managers to address interview options that involve staff

- Provide staff with sample questions that prompt prospective hires to verbalize their skills, rather than having them show a certification card

- Use representatives from the human resources department to educate nurse managers on liability concerns during the interview process, such as those related to discrimination

It is important to help the nurse manager understand that decisions to hire or not to hire will directly affect retention of the staff already on the team. Teaching and guiding them through a process to develop these skills will reveal to them that anyone can look good on paper, but being able to function within the team will only be revealed through skilled interviewing.

Strategies to make time for staff

Almost all nurse managers want to spend more time with their staff, but they have so many responsibilities that they have trouble finding the time. This situation leaves the nurses on the floor with the perception that managers are too busy pushing papers in their offices to spend time with them and do not see what they have to deal with. Time management is always a popular topic at meetings for managers, and although nurse managers often get some training in this area, many people tend to go back to habits they are comfortable with. These old habits are usually the obstacles that prevent managers from using their time effectively.

Manager's support vital to morale

When you talk with staff about what makes them stay at their job, a common response is "my manager." Staff are happy when they feel that their manager respects their contributions and makes time for them. Managers receive satisfaction when they know they are directly responsible for some of the successes in their areas.

All nurse managers must develop an understanding of staff perceptions and how staff relate their importance in the overall picture to how much time their manager spends with them. Develop managers to understand this concept and then to ask themselves how they can change this perception. Many opportunities present themselves at your regular manager meetings, so consider this topic for discussion amongst the nurse manager peer group.

Now is also a good time to look at what you spend time discussing at these meetings. Save the memo reading for another time, and focus on leadership development topics. Start the discussion with suggestions for the nurse manager to consider, such as,

- be available at shift changes several times per week. This doesn't have to be a formal arrangement—just be available.

- schedule to meet with a different staff person one day a week for coffee or sit with them at lunchtime. Pre-schedule and post this information so staff can look forward to it.

- keep a Rolodex file or computer file with each staff person's particulars related to their personal life. When you make time to take someone aside and ask how his or her ill family member is doing, you show that you actually care.

- set up a calendar that lists each staff member's birthday. At the beginning of the month, sign one large card with everyone's name on it and post it in the department.

- post dates and times when you will have an "open door" for anyone who needs to talk. Be sure to stagger the times so all shifts can benefit.

When considering ways to help managers and leaders with their staff's development, ask yourself how you may be affecting retention:

- Have you developed your own goals for each of the managers that report to you?

- How can you personally affect retention of managers?

- Are you willing to change some of your unrealistic expectations of the managers?

- Can you commit, every day, to demonstrating the very behavior, professionalism, and support of the mission that you expect to see from the managers?

- Are you willing to invest time and resources into creating effective processes that enhance the retention of the nurse managers?

You are in a pivotal position not only to develop the managers and the roles they play but also to create processes that retain managers effectively. Those you successfully develop and retain are our administrative healthcare leaders of the future. Feel good about who is going to be leading the way tomorrow by developing the nurse manager today.

Chapter 4

EMPLOYEE- AND FAMILY-FRIENDLY POLICIES AND PROGRAMS

Learning objectives

After reading this chapter, the participant should be able to

- discuss strategies that promote an employee-friendly workplace
- discuss program examples that leave a perception with staff that their employer is family-friendly

Create an environment of care, concern, and respect

A vital part of recruitment and retention is to create a work environment that is employee- and family-friendly. Before you can begin to develop these policies and programs, make sure you are working in a culture that acknowledges and demonstrates care and concern for collegial interests and welfare. Lead through example by interacting with each of your colleagues and peers in a respectful and positive manner at all times.

Encourage positive relationships by taking the time to listen to and learn about the people with whom you work. Know their life priorities and motivators. Learn their children's names and where they're going to school. Ask about their pets. Develop a "significant other" bulletin board, and allow staff to bring photos for display. Include a key at the bottom, identifying the staff member and whether the photo is of a child, parent, partner, pet, or friend.

Treat each person as an individual

Be open-minded and don't make assumptions. When a colleague asks for a special scheduling need, don't respond with "we can't do that here." Discuss the positives and negatives, and if there are concerns, ask the person making the request to do some research. Be willing to explore new options.

Enliven people's days by posting motivational or inspirational quotes on your unit. Clip cartoons and humorous stories that you know relate to a colleague's interest. Begin or end staff meetings by asking everyone to share something positive they experienced in the last week.

Look for positive behaviors in your colleagues and tell them as soon as you can what you saw and how impressed you were with them. In addition, although it may be a more difficult task, talk with colleagues about behaviors you observe that need to be corrected. When a group is asked, "How many would inform a colleague that he or she has bad breath?" only a few will raise their hands. But when asked whether they had bad breath they would want a colleague to tell them, almost everyone in the room raises his or her hand. What this illustrates is that almost all of us are approachable and willing to hear how we can improve, if that approach is done in a thoughtful, encouraging manner. The first step to improving coworker behavior can be daunting, but it is important to take it anyway.

Evaluating employees' needs before creating policies

Although vacation, annual leave, health and dental insurance, and retirement planning have become standard benefits for most healthcare organizations, those seeking to meet the evolving needs of their employees and families should consider several additional benefits and programs.

How to judge employee needs

One of the key elements to success with any employee- or family-oriented program is to know the needs of staff and their families. You can gather this data with a survey and simply hope that you get responses from the majority of people who have the greatest need, or you can use your best resource—the staff who work with you. Form a committee made up of people who know the details and needs of staff members and their families.

Ensure diverse representation on this committee

The members of the committee or task force should include

- staff level employees from all shifts and various types of positions
- employees from diverse age groups
- a balance of male and female employees
- the cultural diversity present in your staff
- staff who do and do not have a need for such programs
- representatives from the mid-level management and top management group
- representatives from personnel or human resources

For workplace enhancement programs to be successful, they must have direct commitment and support from the organization. Both can be accomplished with a clear written statement from senior management that sends a message to all employees that the organization believes in the program and encourages staff and their families to take advantage of what will be offered. Employees must believe the statement is sincere and not feel that they are just being pacified because staff at the hospital down the road got a pay raise and they didn't.

Some tips to consider in helping the committee plan and develop programs include the following:

- Consider rotating members of the committee on an annual basis
- Have clear written objectives and a timeline for what you want them to accomplish
- Give them the resources they need to meet their goals
- Make sure that members of top management are available to sit in on meetings occasionally
- Require written policies for which staff qualify for these programs and how
- Have a process developed to evaluate the effectiveness of each program
- Collect data on frequency usage of each program
- Before enacting any programs charge committee members with educating all of the managers about the programs, rules, policies, etc.

Promote the programs

The best employee- and family-friendly programs cannot help if no one accesses them. Therefore, start a marketing campaign for what you will be offering. Get the word out through word of mouth, e-mail notifications, newsletters, posters, brochures, mailings to employees' homes, and promotional activities at annual employee functions.

Employee assistance programs

Many organizations offer employee assistance programs (EAP), which may be as basic as offering a toll-free hotline for crisis issues or as extensive as counseling for parents and their teenage children. Private companies offer these services to organizations that do not want to be involved in hiring and overseeing the staff that run these programs. Some healthcare organizations want a more "hands on" approach, so they hire staff and are involved with the specifics of the day-to-day operations. Note that the employee assistance program's success will relate directly to how sure staff are that the information is kept confidential. You may want to consider options that include allowing employees to seek appointments on their own for referrals to private counselors. The program could offer monthly training on relationships, addictions, and other problem issues, and it even could assist employees who are in financial turmoil and need temporary assistance. In addition, managers should be able to refer staff to receive counseling from the EAP personnel, should the staff member continue to display unacceptable behaviors.

Manager's role in promoting the employee assistance program

Employees in need of help or in a crisis within their family structure often forget that this service is available to them. Once they finish their orientation process, they tend not to hang onto handbooks and other brochures that explain benefits and free services. Therefore, management should step in to remind staff of these types of services and consider offering it to employees as an option when behavior issues arise. Managers also must trust that the program is strictly confidential; otherwise, they will be unable to reassure staff that it is.

EAP programs may offer numerous benefits

With an active, reputable employee assistance program, your organization not only helps retain valuable staff but also has a wonderful recruiting tool. With so many family challenges in today's world, there is nothing wrong with asking for professional help to get the family unit back on target. Design your employee assistance brochures with targeted services that people feel comfortable talking about, instead of simply highlighting services for domestic violence victims and addictions. Although your employees need to know you offer all these services, the enticement for the program lies in services such as

- financial counseling

- counseling for children, especially teenagers
- classes on negotiating with teens, coping with teens, addressing
  eating disorders, etc.
- marriage retreats
- referrals for employees interested in adopting children
- classes on managing time within the family
- classes for children of divorced parents

On-site health clinics and wellness centers

Another employee and family program that can be of great assistance and can be perceived as a wonderful benefit is a health clinic. Such clinics operate during specific hours and days of the week and are good resources for staff or their immediate family members for minor healthcare needs. Clinics deter employees from using the emergency room as a resource.

Wellness centers offer prevention advice

Another option is to have a wellness center that focuses on primary prevention. More organizations are helping employees maintain physical and emotional wellness by providing an on-site or off-site fitness center, a fitness trainer, a nutritional counselor, and wellness incentives.

Additionally, invest in your employees' health by working toward a no-lift or minimal-lift work environment. Investment in lift-assistive devices to prevent back and joint injuries can be recouped through savings in worker compensation and absenteeism reduction.

Offer a wide variety of benefit options

As well as vacation, medical, and dental benefits, consider offering employees a pre-tax benefit plan, which can provide a variety of pre-tax benefits through an employer-managed plan that can be created under U.S. federal tax law. Certain medical, child care, and adult care expenditures can be paid with these pre-tax dollars. Normally, a pre-tax portion of each paycheck is paid into a reimbursement account and, as eligible expenses are paid, the employee is reimbursed for them.

Some federal employees are allowed seven days in addition to annual or sick leave to serve as bone marrow or organ donors. Other organizations offer leave-sharing programs, whereby fellow employees can donate accumulated leave time to a colleague who may have exhausted his or her own allotment.

Some organizations provide up to $4,000 to assist employee families going through the adoption process. The employees are also granted maternal and paternal leave to promote mother-child and father-child bonding.

Some organizations even allow employees to bring pets to the workplace. Although that my not be possible in direct care settings, some hospitals are negotiating pet health insurance purchase plans and rates for their staff.

Flexible work arrangements

Be open to flexible work arrangements that will meet the needs of both your employees and your organization. By keeping an open mind and exploring different options, you can improve staff satisfaction and retention.

Temporary part time. Some staff may choose to always work part time, but consider options that allow full-time staff to temporarily work part time. This option should be mutually agreed upon by employee and unit manager, but it may be helpful on a short-term basis in times of personal or family crises, or even upon returning from a break.

Job sharing. Allowing and encouraging job sharing, where appropriate, will give part-time flexibility to staff who want it. Under such an arrangement, full-time job responsibilities, duties, hours, and pay can be divided among two or more employees.

Consider non-traditional options

Flextime. Flextime is becoming increasingly popular in the corporate world, and some hospitals are successfully adapting the concept. Some hospitals allow nurses with small children to begin work later in the day so they can drop their children off at school. They work through the day, and in the afternoon, they pick the children up from school, spend quality time with their children and significant other over dinner, and then return to work for a few additional hours. With care, you can develop a flextime policy that allows employees within a team or on an individual basis to choose their own start and finish times.

Compressed work weeks. Although some studies question the safety of working 12-hour shifts, many healthcare employees enjoy the ability to compress their workweek into three or four 12-hour days per week. Likewise, straight weekend or weekend-option schedules are attractive to some healthcare professionals. Consider a variety of shifts, such as eight, 10, and 12 hours, but analyze safety and quality indicators closely so as not to sacrifice either in the name of employee friendliness.

Schedules that coincide with school terms. Another option for employees with school-age children may be to create a work schedule that coincides with your local school term. The term is usually nine months with summers off, but it may be throughout the year if your schools use year-round schedules.

Telecommuting and teleworking. Although nursing is a direct care service, consider tasks that can be completed via computer or telecommunication links to your organization. There may be positions where all or part of the hours can be completed from home.

Carry over leave time. Provide flexibility in allowing staff to carry annual leave into the next calendar year. It should be mutually agreed upon by the manager and employee, but such an arrangement may be helpful in certain situations such as travel abroad.

Employment breaks. Some employees may be interested in taking longer breaks. Consider developing a policy that allows those who have been with you for longer than twelve months to be able to request up to a one-year employment break. Paid employment with another employer would not be taken during this period, and you would assure the individual that, upon return, a job of equal status within your organization would be provided. Personal reasons that might warrant interest in this benefit include a prolonged illness in the family, care of a parent, charity work, or world travel.

Self-scheduling. This option allows unit staff to schedule their time based on parameters negotiated by the unit manager and staff. It promotes satisfaction and autonomy among employees.

Phased retirement. This option allows older employees to retire gradually by reducing full-time hours over a period of years. As demand for healthcare professionals increases, some states are enacting policy to remove retirement penalties and work limits to allow qualifying employees to receive full retirement benefits and continue to work full time.

Programs that save employees time

Many of these programs ask, what can you do to make life easier for the employee? Any time you can answer this question with a program or service, you have created a recruitment and retention tool.

Everyone wants more time, so help your employees find time for activities they value. Providing the following types of services gives employees more time with their families when they are not at work:

- The third Wednesday of each month, staff can call the local grocery store and reserve a complete cooked dinner, for a special price. They pick it up that day between specified hours.

- The local dry cleaner has an area in the hospital where staff can leave their clothes for dry cleaning and pick them back up the next work day. Payment is prearranged through the employee's credit card, so the hospital does not have to deal with financial transactions.

- An arrangement is made with the local optical shop for all employees and their immediate family members to receive a discount on eye exams and frames or contact lenses.

- A local oil change company picks up employees' cars from the hospital parking lot and returns them after an oil change. Payment can also be handled through the employee's credit card.

Other employee- and family-friendly programs

Child care. Some hospitals provide on-site child care services, and others negotiate rates and openings with local child care agencies. Having child care options can benefit a large portion of your staff, and worker satisfaction increases when parents are happy with their child care arrangements.

Adult care. You may be surprised at the number of employees who are primary care provides for their parents or older relatives. These employees may be more interested in adult care services as a benefit.

Help with partner's employment search. Consider providing assistance with an employment search of a spouse or partner of a candidate or current employee with a partner opportunities program.

Seminars. Make an effort to meet other needs of your employees by providing "brown-bag" or evening seminars on a variety of family issues. Survey your staff to determine their interests and what they may find most helpful or interesting.

Showing employees that you value them

Make a commitment to demonstrating to employees that they are valued.

The power of everyday surprises

Regardless of age and occupation, many people love surprises. It is the element of the unexpected and the fact that someone took the time to think of it that make it special.

If you develop leadership skills in your managers by teaching this concept, you empower them with simple employee-friendly ideas. The size of the surprise does not necessarily relate to how happy it makes the person on the receiving end. Surprises do not have to be attached to rewards, although they can and should be when appropriate. Surprises are not simply about celebrating a birthday in the department.

Simple surprises
- The manager takes the assignment of the nurse who has the longest tenure. After the manager gets the nurse's patient report, the nurse is sent home for the shift with pay and a large card thanking him or her for his or her commitment to the patients and the organization.

- At shift change, surprise staff by stationing top-level management outside with buckets of soap, sponges, and hoses to wash employees' cars before they go home.

- The director of nurses arrives unexpectedly on a nursing unit and works side by side for the entire shift with a newly hired nurse.

- The CEO of the organization calls a nurse manager in the morning and invites him or her to lunch that day to brainstorm and share ideas about improving patient care.

What employees really want

Although some employee- and family-friendly policies may be fairly easy to implement, organizations must not lose sight of the bigger picture. In 2004, Accenture Consulting[1] surveyed 1,501 recent college graduates to find out what they wanted most from their prospective new employers. The results revealed that training and compensation were at the top of the graduate's wish list.

What they desired most from an employer

Training programs	71%
Fair compensation	61%
Flexible schedules	59%
Approachable and available management	55%
Ethical management	48%
Mentorship programs	45%
Social gatherings/events	30%
Discounts at local shops	23%
Telecommuting	16%

These results remind us that although employee- and family-friendly programs are important, they should not be developed to replace other vital qualities employees need from their employers, such as trust, ethics, training, and development.

References

1. Amanda C. Kooser, "Workplace 2005," *Entrepreneur* (February 2005): 58.

Chapter 5

DEVELOPING PROFESSIONAL MODELS OF CARE

Learning objectives

After reading this chapter, the participant should be able to

- identify the components of professional models of care
- discuss the benefits of professional models of care

Professional models of care promote retention

Professional models of patient care delivery are constantly changing and improving. Employees in any profession want to work in an organization that provides a great product or service, and nurses in healthcare settings are no different. They want to work in settings that provide great patient care.

Health consumers have high expectations for healthcare delivery systems, and it is only right that they should expect safe, quality, individualized care. To address patient expectations for quality care, healthcare systems must develop nursing care delivery systems that encourage, support, and develop nurse autonomy and decision-making.

Allow nurses to practice to the best of their ability

Employers should construct and implement systems that allow nurses to practice within their full scope of practice. Practice policies and procedures should be based on nursing practice standards and evidence-based outcomes. Employers must recognize, through support of clinical research and nurse-directed care improvements, that nurses contribute knowledge and expertise to quality patient care and patient outcomes. The positive influence of professional models of care on nurse retention is well documented through Magnet hospital research studies.[1]

Strong nursing leadership

Managers play an integral role in creating a unit culture of quality care and workplace improvement. Therefore, hire qualified, well-prepared nurse managers capable of fulfilling management functions and roles. Provide support and encouragement for nurse managers through programs and policies. Develop a comprehensive list of manager competencies, including such basics as

- adherence to ethics and practice standards
- effective communication and interpersonal skills
- conflict resolution
- decision-making
- problem solving
- delegation
- human resource management
- financial and budget management
- provision of staff evaluations and performance appraisals

Also inquire about their abilities to demonstrate broader manager competencies, such as
- caring for self, patients, and staff
- implementing quality improvement processes
- negotiation and conflict resolution
- promoting collaborative interdisciplinary relationships
- developing staff
- systems and administrative theories
- financial resource monitoring
- human resource monitoring
- political savvy

- research utilization and implementation
- policy development
- strategic planning

Help managers look critically at their skills and develop a program for self-improvement. You'll want to groom staff nurses to help with operational functions whenever possible to allow managers to focus on these broader management and leadership skills.

In a culture constantly seeking improvements, managers do not only need to manage—they also need to lead. As a manager, you must manage resources and work with your staff to remove barriers to quality care, but as a leader, you must improve your self-knowledge regarding areas of strength and areas you can improve. Thus, becoming a leader involves developing strategic skills that help position your unit for a successful future. It includes taking risks, incorporating creative ways of group problem-solving, and improving patient care. Leadership requires you to develop coaching, mentoring, and grooming skills. It includes shaping and sharing compelling messages that inspire and encourage staff nurses to provide organizational policy development, strategic planning, and operational decision-making in an effort to improve patient care. In a professional work environment, nurse managers and leaders make sure that nursing is an integral part of any organizational committee that governs policy and operational decision-making.

Nurse-directed patient care

Establish unit and organizational cultures that encourage and demand nurse-directed care. In professional practice models, nurses make autonomous decisions within their scopes of practice and control care-delivery standards in the practice environment. Nurses are responsible and accountable for all nursing practices. They establish practice standards, set patient care goals, make decisions concerning managing and monitoring patient care, and measure patient outcomes. Work with your staff and administration to develop and implement policies that mandate nurse authority to control nursing practice by developing nursing care policies.

Review your organizational structure periodically with staff, and discuss the impact of communication and decision-making at the point of care. Use staff meetings to share examples of decisions made by nurses on your unit that directly influenced positive patient outcomes.

You might even begin staff meetings by asking staff to share how their decisions made a difference in patient care and improved satisfaction. You also can ask them to share a decision that made them feel uneasy or uncertain, and either confirm their actions or ask fellow staff to discuss how they would have reacted to that type of situation. Reaffirm your commitment to nurse decision-making at the point of care, and assess staff needs for continuing education programs that promote self-development in decision-making and leadership skills.

Shared governance

Shared governance is an integral component of several professional practice models. These models essentially promote nurse empowerment by including direct care nurses on organizational committees and in administrative decision-making. They use a democratic process based upon the combined expertise of a group of nurse professionals. With shared governance, organizations establish several committees or councils to provide collective decision-making and may include one or more of the following:

1. Coordinating council

Usually chaired by the chief nursing officer, membership includes staff nurses and nurse managers. Its purpose is to develop the organization's strategic plan and recommend agenda items to other appropriate councils.

2. Nurse practice or clinical practice council

Usually chaired by a senior staff nurse, membership includes staff nurses representing individual units or service lines. The council develops patient care policy and standards based on the strategic plan. Interdepartmental and interdisciplinary concerns may be shared in this forum. New technology may be reviewed and compared prior to hospitalwide purchase and use.

3. Quality/performance improvement council

Chaired by a staff nurse, its goal is to discuss issues and make decisions pertaining to the delivery of quality patient care. The council works to ensure quality care by identifying quality priorities and indicator measurements. It may also be utilized to recognize employee contributions related to quality patient care.

4. Management council

Usually chaired by a nurse manager or leader, this group is responsible for distribution of fiscal resources, staffing, and provides input on hiring practices and decisions.

5. Education council

Usually chaired by a nurse educator or staff nurse. This council promotes professional growth of nurses by identifying continuing-education programs based on competencies needed in various nurse roles.

6. Research council

Chaired by a staff nurse, the research council encourages implementation of research and evidence-based projects in clinical areas.

Having nurses participate in the shared governance structures and councils encourages nurses to be autonomous and accountable decision-makers at the point of care. It also encourages them to practice fully within the scope and professional standards of nursing practice.

Adequate and appropriate staffing

Adequate staffing is another component of professional care models. The adequacy of hospital staffing, in the form of mandated nurse-to-patient ratios, has received much attention in recent years. The goal is to provide cost-effective, quality staff and staffing patterns. Ultimately, staffing decisions must be made by nurses and nurse managers on a moment-by-moment basis. Tools for measuring patient acuity may assist nurses in staffing decisions, but no one acuity measurement system has proven more accurate or effective than others. A nurse may receive the same five patients on two separate shifts, and each can exhibit very different care demands. In addition, care demands can change dramatically within the same work shift. Therefore, staffing decisions must be made by staff nurses and nurse managers as patient needs change at the point of care.

Make sure you are using the right healthcare professional with the correct competencies for providing quality patient care. Plan your staffing patterns to maintain an adequate number of qualified nurses to meet changing acute and complex patient needs.

Staffing options

Always adjust staffing patterns as patient demands change, and encourage employees to make suggestions concerning staffing options. Ask for their thoughts on times when they feel that the unit may be understaffed or overstaffed. Some hospitals are using a mid-shift "huddle" in which nurses and staff nurses gather for a two-minute report on how each staff member is doing. At that point, the charge nurse can reprioritize or change work assignments for the remainder of the shift.

However you make your decisions, promote teamwork and consider strategies that extend the present work force, such as making support services and personnel available to help nurses meet evolving patient care demands. For example, if your staff feel that the unit is understaffed due to multiple admissions/discharges, try placing an extra nurse on the unit to do just admissions and discharges. Some hospitals hire nurses in the admissions office to conduct the admission assessment before patients are transferred to their rooms.

Develop a formal system of evaluation

Develop a formal system for evaluating the effects of staffing patterns and skill mix on patient outcomes. For example, develop a tool that charge nurses use to rate the adequacy of staffing on each shift. However you measure it, make sure that staffing is consistently adequate to provide quality patient care.

Consider hiring advanced practice nurses (e.g., clinical nurse specialists, nurse practitioners, nurse researchers, educators) to ensure delivery of quality patient care. Make those nurses available to support nurses who have less experience. Also help your staff establish unit-wide minimum staffing standards, and use self-scheduling principles to plan work schedules.

Quality improvement processes

Professional work environments are committed to quality improvement, evidence-based practice, and quality patient care. Make sure nurses are incorporated into unit and organizational quality improvement committees, and provide nurses with continuing education, coaching, and role modeling in research and evidence-based practice. Identify expected outcomes with benchmarks for acceptable quality service, and conduct quality outcome measurements to determine your progress. Traditionally, quality improvement processes have been applied almost exclusively to improving patient care, but be sure to apply the same processes to improving your workplace culture and environment.

Report your results

Provide quality care outcomes or indicators to your quality council or nurse practice council to recommend practice improvements and address concerns. Establish a utilization review system to conduct analysis and correction of patient care and safety concerns and issues.

Providing interdisciplinary forums will encourage discussion of collaborative strategies for improving patient care and eliminating duplication of services among disciplines. Develop processes for immediate reporting of unsafe or poor care, and implement a system by which employees can recognize and reward colleagues who deliver quality patient care.

Building competent teams

Helping your staff with self-improvement can be as simple as asking one of your experienced staff nurses to initiate and lead a journal club. The leader of the club selects an article, makes copies or posts it on your unit bulletin board, and has members of the club meet for 15–30 minutes to discuss the findings that apply to your unit. The discussion might occur at the beginning of a staff meeting, and other staff nurses could be allowed to suggest articles for the group to review. Such a club is a great strategy for applying the latest research findings to the practice setting, and it helps your staff to keep up with the latest skills and competencies.

Valuing colleagues

Help employees understand the value of individual contributions to quality patient care. Discuss the team effort required and establish a culture of mutual valuing and respect. Help your staff understand that each individual contributes specific skills and competencies and that each is important. Cafeteria workers, housekeeping staff, nursing assistants, nurses, nurse managers, and physicians all contribute to quality patient care.

Develop a "We Care" rather than a "Me Care" patient safety and quality care culture. Help staff understand that the delivery of quality care requires more than just holding oneself accountable for doing the right things—it also requires healthcare professionals to make sure our healthcare systems help all personnel to do the right things, leaving little or no room for error. Help staff develop policies and systems that encourage them to deliver safe, quality, ethical, and error-free care.

With the stress of a healthcare work environment and the diverse personalities, opinions, and competencies among personnel, conflict is inevitable. Therefore, develop formal processes for dealing with it. Establish behavior standards or a professional conduct code that includes zero tolerance for rude or demeaning behavior, and make sure staff are aware of the policies. These policies should require immediate counseling by managers or supervisors for internal personnel and by the chief nursing officer or chief executive officer for external personnel (e.g., physicians, paramedics, or visitors).

Measuring benefits of professional models of care

Using components and principles of professional models of care can improve staff retention and quality patient care. Doing so makes healthcare safer, as demonstrated by lower error rates, and improves quality of care delivery, as evidenced by higher patient satisfaction scores. Other benefits of incorporating professional models of care are that the retention of nurses and healthcare personnel improves through lower turnover rates, lower vacancy rates, and higher retention rates. Staff morale is improved and demonstrated by higher employee satisfaction scores.

References

1. M. McClure and A. Hinshaw, *Magnet Hospitals Revisited: Attraction and Retention of Professional Nurses* (Washington, DC: American Nurses Publishing, 2002).

Chapter 6

IMPLEMENTING QUALITY WORKPLACE IMPROVEMENT SYSTEMS

Learning objectives

After reading this chapter, the participant should be able to

- identify ways to implement quality workplace improvement systems
- evaluate the results of implementing quality workplace improvement systems

The need for quality improvement systems

Quality improvement processes and systems dramatically improve patient care outcomes. It is in the best interest of every hospital and healthcare delivery system to develop patient care standards and systems that consistently improve patient safety and care. It is also in the best interest of healthcare employers to implement quality workplace improvement processes and systems to create a workplace culture and environment that attracts and retains excellent healthcare professionals.

In such a quality workplace, nurse managers, administration, and staff support a quality work environment. They develop standards and systems for sustaining a quality workplace. Nurse leaders receive essential data and information, have authority and accountability, and are integrally involved in decisions that affect the workplace environment.

First steps in developing quality improvement systems

When beginning a program, first ensure that administrator, manager, and staff performance evaluations include the criteria for creating a quality workplace. Also incorporate workplace improvement criteria into staff nurse and other healthcare employee performance appraisals.

Establish clear goals for workplace excellence. Develop systems that not only meet Occupational Safety and Health Administration standards but also exceed regulatory workplace safety standards. In a service-delivery profession, your employees are among your most valuable assets.

Create a workplace environment council

Includes nurses and other employees on committees responsible for ensuring worker safety and illness prevention. For example, you can use your management council to identify and make recommendations concerning workplace improvements or establish a workplace environment council. One of the group's responsibilities might be to evaluate the purchase of products or systems that promote employee safety.

Although ensuring patient and employee safety may be a basic goal of these committees, a loftier goal would be to create a workplace environment that fosters employee wellness, engagement, and commitment. Therefore, ask the committee to develop strategies that promote physical, emotional, spiritual, professional, and social wellness of your staff. It could make recommendations concerning meaningful work and develop policies and programs that promote employee engagement and commitment—and an engaged and committed employee is a loyal employee.

A workplace environment council will focus on prevention strategies to decrease illness, injury, stress, and accidents among employees. Consider placing at least one member on the human resources committee that reviews compensation and benefits.

Councils also can collect data on employee satisfaction and make evidence-based recommendations based upon employees' needs and interests. The council might recommend a no-lift or minimal-lift policy. They also might develop an initiative to prevent workplace violence and provide support for employees who experience violence. The council could set safety and security quality improvement goals and conduct root cause analysis on incidents involving employees.

Quality workplace improvement principles

Several principles are helpful when considering quality workplace improvements.

Focus on the employee

The ultimate customers of any healthcare delivery organization are the patients, but the most important internal customers are your employees. If you care for your employees, they will care for your patients. You cannot deliver patient care without healthcare professionals, and each has unique needs, wants, and motivators. Thus, just as hospitals have established systems and processes to deliver individualized, customized patient care, they must develop systems and processes to provide individualized, customized employee care.

Understand work culture as systems and processes

When you look at the complete picture of a workplace culture and environment, it can seem incomprehensible and overwhelming. Therefore, take one thing at a time, and analyze specific systems and processes. For example, identify communication processes that occur among staff, such as nurse to nurse, or nurse to nursing assistant. Talk with your staff to ascertain what needs to be improved first.

Also seek to improve collaboration among and between staff, such as nurses, nursing assistants, staff on different shifts, and so on. Focus your efforts to improve one system or process at a time, and begin with the areas that are causing most dissatisfaction among your staff.

Teamwork

Include as many of your staff in the improvement discussions as you can. Ask for their thoughts, ideas, and assistance in putting improvements in place. Each has a vested interest in improving the workplace, and because each is a frontline employee, each can contribute significant insight and expertise. As a manager, define parameters or limits for workplace improvement discussions, but make sure that you use their helpful recommendations and suggestions. Remind your staff that workplace improvements should benefit the entire healthcare team.

Focus on the use of data

Help staff understand the power of data. When a particular issue is raised, ask the staff to document it for a week or so to determine how often the type of incident actually occurs. For example, if linens are late arriving on the unit, have the charge nurses document how often it occurs before you decide whether to take corrective action. If staff report an increase in belligerent visitors, ask them to document the time of day it occurs. Upon analysis, you might find that the incidents are occurring during change of shift, so you can look at strategies to decrease some of the chaos that occurs at that time. You'll want your workplace improvements to be evidence-based, and data provides that evidence.

Key steps to improvement

Establishing where to begin your quality workplace improvement is the first challenge.

Begin with what's causing the most pain

Identify what's causing your staff the most concern or pain. Ask your staff to develop a list of workplace issues they would like to see improved, and help them to prioritize and select issues to be addressed. Be aware that if your staff have not participated in this type of process, you may want to begin with a few issues where you can demonstrate quick successes. For example, instead of beginning by trying to improve employee parking, begin by contracting with a local dry cleaner to provide pick-up and delivery service. Once they have a few successes under their belt, you can help them tackle more challenging workplace issues, such as improving nurse-physician relations or collaboration with other units. Use data from your employee satisfaction survey, exit interviews, or staff discussions to identify workplace improvement issues.

Develop a workplace improvement council

Although retention is everyone's responsibility, you'll need to establish a committee or council to focus on workplace improvements. Some organizations use a recruitment and retention committee, which usually focuses on recruitment and retention strategies, but the workplace council discussed earlier is often a better option because its goal is to provide a quality workplace, which would enhance both recruitment and retention.

Collect and analyze workplace data and information

It is imperative that you collect a variety of workplace data, and at times you'll want to implement research and outcomes studies. Establish systems that provide constant feedback from your employees. Don't collect data for the sake of collecting data. Only collect what you need, but give thoughtful consideration to data sources that will help you identify workplace improvement trends and issues. Use evidence-based decision-making to identify areas for change and improvement.

Exit interviews

When employees leave your organization, collect exit interview data in a consistent, anonymous manner so they can tell you the real reasons they're leaving. Most employees do not want to decrease their chances of being rehired if needed, so make sure they feel that they can be truthful in their responses. Managers should not administer the exit interview but instead should have it administered by computer, conducted in the human resources office, or outsourced to a third party.

Performance appraisals

Annual performance appraisals are an ideal time to collect employee ideas on workplace improvements. You're probably already using performance appraisals to determine competency training needed for your unit. Consider including competencies that relate to interpersonal communication and interdisciplinary collaboration. You also might ask each employee to share the top three things he or she likes most about working on your unit and the top three things he or she likes least about working there. If you tally your responses, you'll get an idea of what features are valued by your staff and are working, and make sure the needs of your staff continue to be met. An analysis of the items they like least will help you focus on areas for workplace improvements.

Incremental interviews

Incremental interviews are used when you learn that an employee is considering leaving your unit and you'd like to retain him or her. This interview can provide helpful information for workplace improvements, but its main focus is to prevent a quality staff member from leaving. You certainly can ask what they like or do not like about working there, but the main question you'll ask is, "What can we do to keep you here?" You'll also want to spend time identifying their career goals and discussing options you can provide on your unit to help them achieve those goals.

Individualized measurements

There may be times you will want to conduct individualized measurements of specific workplace issues. For example, you may wish to evaluate employee levels of stress. Particularly when the patient census is high, measure levels of employee stress and identify stressors in the work environment. You also might determine the types of strategies that help relieve stress for your staff.

Use appreciative inquiry

Collect data through appreciative inquiry by asking your staff to identify what your organization is doing right, rather than what it is not. Although it can be helpful to make improvements in an organization, appreciative inquiry helps to identify what's working well. Rather than focusing on what is wrong with a system, this theory advises organizations to focus on strengths and capabilities to achieve improvement goals. Ask your staff to share workplace improvement success stories. If you're focusing on improving interpersonal communication, have staff share communication behaviors they observed during the workday that promoted positive outcomes. The goal is to verbalize positive behaviors that you would like other staff to replicate. Appreciative inquiry has helped several healthcare systems improve patient satisfaction, and it holds great promise to do the same for employee satisfaction.

Focus groups

Bring together groups of eight to ten staff to focus on specific issues. If you're attempting to develop strategies to retain mature, experienced nurses, invite a group of nurses who are fifty and older from different units and shifts to identify incentives, benefits, and work improvements that would encourage them to work longer. You might decide to hold a focus group for each shift.

To get consistent group responses, develop a script with questions to use with each group. Response data and information from the groups can be documented, tallied, and analyzed to identify priority issues and strategies.

Monitor employee satisfaction

More and more employers understand the need to monitor employee satisfaction. Healthcare delivery is an employee-intensive service, so it is especially vital for employers to retain staff. Some hospitals are outsourcing employee satisfaction surveys and data analysis. Others have developed an in-house employee satisfaction survey tool. Either is fine, as long as it provides unbiased trends and findings pertaining to employee satisfaction. Use employee satisfaction findings to help identify areas and issues for workplace improvement.

Considering change and improvement

Upon reviewing findings and trends from multiple sources of workplace data, or after hearing a workplace issue verbalized by numerous staff members, you will begin to think, "Maybe we should do something about this." It's at that moment that you must consider whether it is worth the effort to make the change or improvement, or whether it is better to maintain the status quo. Here's a process that will help you make that decision.

1. Identify what must improve

This step may sound redundant, but you must determine what needs to improve. For example, let's say that your employee-satisfaction survey identifies that nurses feel nurse-physician interactions need major improvement. As a nurse manager, you may already hold insight into the particulars of the issue, and the employee satisfaction findings only validate your earlier suspicions. But let's say you had no idea that nurse-physician interactions needed improvement. To determine what actually needs to improve, you might talk with some of your nurses or physicians to gather more in-depth information. You might even hold a focus group with nurses and one with physicians to gather input. Are the negative interactions coming from one-on-one discussions? Does it relate to calling physicians in the middle of the night? Or is it a professional trust issue? Your goal is to determine what must improve.

2. Analyze and understand the problem

Help your workplace improvement group analyze and understand the problem. Make sure they have all available data and information, and allow time to discuss, dissect, and process problem scenarios. Ask them to identify specific systems and processes that require improvement, and require them to recommend desired outcomes.

3. Consider and develop

Consider what changes will improve the problem, and develop strategies that accomplish your desired outcomes. Brainstorming can be a useful technique for developing strategies. Ask your employees to blurt out any ideas, no matter how wacky or way out, in a 10-minute period. Ask one staff member to write the ideas on a flip chart as they are suggested. The only rule is that no one is allowed to judge another staff member's idea. After the ideas are documented, encourage the group to select the top three strategies for further discussion and consideration.

4. Test and implement

Consider testing your thoughts and recommendations to see whether they yield improvements. Once your staff have determined a best option, develop plans to test the strategy to see whether it provides desired outcomes. Then you and your staff can decide whether to abandon, modify, or permanently implement the solution.

A model for testing change in the workplace

Plan

Develop a plan for the change. Consider the impact of the change on patient care, workplace, and employee outcomes. Identify methods for measuring your desired outcomes. Make sure you and your staff communicate the pilot test for change to all employees affected by the change.

Pilot test

Establish start and completion dates, and test the change. Collect data and document the results of the change. Continue to monitor the outcomes.

Analyze results

Review data, and realistically evaluate positive or negative effects of the change. Verify your methods and results to make sure they are accurate.

Implement change

Modify, abandon, or implement the change. Develop a process to monitor outcomes consistently and consider implementing the improvement in your workplace.

Examples of successful quality workplace improvement initiatives

The following examples are successful workplace improvements implemented in hospitals across the country. You and your staff will need to work closely and diligently to address evolving issues in your own workplace environment. Your goal is to create an excellent workplace environment that engages your employees to deliver excellent patient care.

1. Nurse-developed intranet that provides easy access to nursing council activities, nursing news, and nursing procedures. Alaska Native Medical Center: Anchorage

2. Preceptor directed internship program to facilitate novice to expert skill development. Sarasota Memorial Hospital: Sarasota, FL

3. Nurse managers responsible for one unit and report directly to the vice president of patient care services. Children's Mercy Hospital and Clinics: Kansas City, MO

4. Friends of Nursing Program recognizes excellence in nursing practice, education, and research. Lehigh Valley Hospital and Health Network: Allentown and Bethlehem, PA

5. Nurses collaborate with human resources on compensation, recruitment, retention, and special pay incentives. Seton Medical Center: Austin, TX

6. Local university provides on-site BSN and MSN programs. Community Medical Center: Toms River, NJ

7. Fund for Nursing Excellence supports educational/professional development, recognition of outstanding accomplishments, and clinical projects/nursing studies that promote excellent practice. Holmes Regional Medical Center and Palm Bay Community Hospital: Melbourne and Palm Bay, FL

8. Graduate Nurse Orientation Success in Specialties program progresses new graduates into specialty of choice. High Point Regional Hospital: High Point, NC

9. "Medical Excellence" program promotes excellence in competence, citizenship and leadership, continuous quality improvement, service response, education, integrity, and behavior. Morton Plant Mease Healthcare: Clearwater, FL

10. Annual measurement of nurses' perceptions of autonomy, control over practice, and strength of collaborative relationships with physicians and other members of the healthcare team. Massachusetts General Hospital: Boston

11. Established chief retention officer with unit-level retention committees. Medical City Dallas Hospital and the North Texas Hospital for Children at Medical City: Dallas

12. Assistant Clinical Nurse Manager mentors and develops new staff. Wake Forest University Baptist Medical Center: Winston-Salem, NC

13. Nurse researchers and clinical nurse specialists serve as adjunct faculty at area colleges and universities. Miami Children's Hospital: Miami, FL

14. Resource nurse on each unit with no patient assignments—assists with admissions/discharges, procedures, internal transport, seriously ill patients, and patient assignments. Children's Mercy Hospital and Clinics: Kansas City, MO

Chapter 7

ENSURING INTERDISCIPLINARY COLLABORATION

Learning objectives

After reading this chapter, the participant should be able to

- identify effective methods of promoting collaborative practice between nursing, medicine, and other professional departments
- discuss the benefits when nursing staff actively participate in collaborative systems and processes related to patient care

Lack of collaboration breeds discontent

The nurses on an inpatient neurology unit have all worked together for several years. They feel a strong presence of team support amongst their peers and are encouraged by a manager who uses effective strategies to enhance their work environment. So why are they unhappy? The hospital has negotiated a new contract for neurosurgery services with a larger group from the city hospital about one hour away, and new people have entered the environment. What was a peaceful workplace has become a battlefield.

The situation is a classic example of a non-collaborative environment. The new medical staff showed up at the hospital with unrealistic expectations of the existing staff, and the nursing staff were not involved in the process of changing to a new medical team. The facility took no steps to get the new relationship off to a good start, and the end result was an environment filled with difficult scenarios.

First, the new medical staff requested procedures and supplies that the nurses were unfamiliar with, and the nurses were criticized for not having these supplies. The standing orders from the previous medical team were still being carried out, which left the nursing staff vulnerable when they had to call a doctor at night about an order that the physician had no idea was in place. The nursing staff generally felt inadequate, and the new medical staff perceived them that way.

The importance of collaboration

Such situations do not make for the best patient care, nor do they create an environment that enhances recruitment and retention.

When you are ready to establish goals to enhance collaborative practice, begin with a process that causes staff to take a step back and truly understand what collaborative practices are about. One way to initiate this process is to have the medical staff, nursing staff, and other professional departments, such as respiratory therapy and pharmacy, participate in a survey that asks questions such as the following:

1. What does the term "collaborative practice" mean to you?
2. Do you feel that by improving collaborative efforts we improve patient care?
3. What are two things you can do to improve/enhance collaborative practice?
4. What are two things other professionals can do to enhance collaborative efforts?
5. Would you be interested in being part of a team that works with administration on a project targeted to improve collaborative practices in our organization?

You can use this survey to begin to educate staff about collaboration by giving them a question that requires them to look at the literal definition of the term. For example:

Which of the following terms are synonyms for collaboration?
Joint, group effort, two-way, relationship, mutual, cooperation, shared, teamwork

This type of exercise reminds people that collaboration is more than co-signing standing orders or serving on the same committee.

Successful collaboration

Managers must lead by example to establish good relationships with coworkers. For example, the respiratory therapy budget is being challenged, and the end result is that some nursing units will be required to administer specific breathing treatments that previously had been administered by respiratory therapy. Using collaborative practice, the managers of these two departments worked together before approaching their staff members. When they were ready to present the change at the staff level, they continued the collaboration process by doing it at a joint staff meeting to show they were working as a team to identify the best approach to this challenge. This scenario reminds us that if managers work in collaboration with other managers, they can much more reasonably expect staff to do so.

Collaboration is facility-wide

When nurses hear the word "collaboration," they often think of the medical staff, due to the frequency of the interaction of nursing and medicine. In contrast, when medical staff hear the word, they often think of working well within their own peer group. Your first step toward improving collaboration may be simply to raise awareness among all employees that all departments and all employees must collaborate in order to provide effective and safe patient care.

Case study: Problem relationships

The new nurse manager had been warned about the ear nose and throat (ENT) specialist who had such a difficult personality that many nurses feared calling him at night. When he stepped off the elevator, nurses would scatter. His behavior was widely known, and in all the years that he had been part of the medical staff, no one had confronted him about his behavior—not even the administrative team.

At the beginning of the day shift, the new manager went onto the unit to see how things had gone on the night shift, and she ran into the ENT physician. She had not yet had the opportunity to meet him, and he caught her off guard. He immediately began a verbal harangue, listing the things "her staff did wrong" and asking, "How could you allow this?"

This was the first management position for the nurse, and she was unprepared for such an abrasive situation. She began to cry and went to her office to hide from him. Her reaction took the physician by surprise, and he left the unit without saying a word. The next day, the nurse manager received flowers from the physician—and an in-person apology. This led to a collaborative discussion between the nurse manager and the physician, in which he revealed that he did not realize how his behavior had been affecting others. The conversation also brought to light some issues related to some legitimate patient care concerns the physician had, which he had been expressing for years but which were ignored due to the lack of relationship between him and the nursing staff.

Challenges of the healthcare environment

The healthcare environment throws many challenges at us as we try to enhance our teams and learn to work more effectively with other departments. These challenges include over-worked and tired staff, high-acuity patients and stressful decision-making environments, and administration's unwillingness to address unacceptable behaviors.

We cannot allow these challenges to be an excuse for not moving forward with collaborative practices. For some organizations, the biggest hurdle may be to get past the concept of "that's the way we've always done it around here."

When we approach the concerns related to lack of communication, teamwork, and mutual goals, there is one thing we know for sure: Most people want what is in the best interest of the patient. When looking at collaborative practice issues, be sure to address patient outcomes. No matter how many interdisciplinary committees you have, they are worth little if you are not improving patient outcomes. Your efforts in every area should always aim to do so.

Leadership's role

Magnet-status hospitals continue to guide us, through their successes, in ensuring that leadership plays a direct role in encouraging and nurturing collaborative practices. By gauging effectiveness and by measuring patient outcomes, we can show with certainty the success of efforts directed at team building and improving communication processes and systems.

Because improving collaboration is an ongoing process that will require leadership oversight and management, develop some working goals to help you manage your efforts in enhancing collaboration:

1. Assess nursing and medical staff perceptions of the current status of collaboration.
2. Ask the organization's leadership staff about their perceptions of the status of collaboration in the organization. Include mid-level managers in this assessment.
3. Identify two successful collaborative efforts that have occurred in the past three years, and review the following:

   • Why were they successful?
   • Is the effort still in progress?
   • Who or what was the motivating force for the success?
   • Were patient outcomes related and, if so, how were they measured?

4. Obtain input from nursing and medical staff on their perception of the top three patient care concerns that need collaborative attention.

5. Compare these results with the responses from the leadership team.

After you have collected information,

   • share responses to survey questions at the next management meeting

   • develop a collaborative improvement team, and have top management appoint people who submitted targeted comments and suggestions on their surveys

   • involve staff responsible for compliance with Joint Commission of Accreditation of Healthcare Organizations (JCAHO) standards and risk management in your improvement processes

   • actively involve newly hired nurses and physicians so that you have staff with fresh perspectives, unhindered by history of events at your organization

   • include the concept of collaborative practice in the orientation process

Case study: Why we work here

Amy has been a nurse on the telemetry floor for three years, and James, a former college classmate, is relocating to her neighborhood and looking for a new job. Amy is located in a large city, so the competition amongst local hospitals for nurses is fierce, with recruitment efforts often solely focused on the amount of money offered in sign-on bonuses.

The department manager on the telemetry unit where Amy works has made it a department standard that all nursing staff be involved in patient care practices, systems, and shared accountabilities. Amy knows that she is part of something special, from the self-scheduling concept on the unit to the committee directed by one of the cardiologists. James asked Amy about what the hospital is really like:

James: "Tell me the real story about what goes on in that unit. I met with the manager yesterday, and you know they all make things sound great.

Amy: "No place is perfect. You learn what becomes really important once you have been out of school and working for a while. But I never thought I would sit on a committee with a cardiologist who actually listened to my ideas about post-cath patients.

Everyone thinks these people can just get out of here once the sheath is pulled, but I told him about some situations we had over here, and he really listened. Working on the right shift is not ideal, but I value this place—knowing that the docs here respect me and my input counts for something means I'll wait for the next day shift opening."

Importance of collaboration in recruitment and retention

This process must not be done only at the top-level of the administration. Instead, it needs to be brought down to the individual department level, where you will see the benefit it brings to nursing recruitment and retention. Creating an environment of mutual collaboration leads not only to improved patient outcomes but also to a positive work experience.

One of the most important aspects of this scenario is that all parties involved realize that their work is making a difference. For example, the cardiologist should receive feedback about the impact he or she is having on nursing recruitment and retention. If you don't share this type of information on a regular basis, you can easily lose some of your best cheerleaders for collaborative practice.

Create collaborative relationships between nurses, medical staff, and other departments

Here are the necessary steps to create and build a collaborative atmosphere:

1. Decide once and for all to stop tolerating unacceptable behavior

Would you want to show up for work or come in to see a patient at 3:00 a.m. if you knew that the person with whom you had to collaborate exhibited behavior that you would not tolerate in your house? Whether it is foul language, rude tone of voice, or negative comments about you or your team, the bottom line is that if you would not tolerate it at home, you should not tolerate it at work.

Nurses Connie Linck and Susan Phillips evaluated the results of such disruptive behavior and found that it caused

- physicians to be distracted when trying to write orders or dictate

- nurses to be distracted drawing up or calculating medication

- patients or families who see or hear the disruptive behavior to have reduced confidence in staff's abilities

- patients and families to have poor perceptions of how medical professionals act and treat one another

- other team members who witnessed the behavior to lose any desire to work with the disruptive people and to shy away from being available to help them out when needed[1]

At home, we put kids in time out for anti-social behavior; at work, we use job descriptions and the mission/vision statement to hold people accountable. Develop policies and procedures and medical staff bylaws that identify your definition of disruptive or unacceptable behaviors. Include strong language that reflects the organization's unwillingness to tolerate these behaviors and what the disciplinary process will be for those who elect not to change.

2. Educate management/employees on appropriate communication methods and tools

This process should begin on the first day of orientation and continue on an annual basis. It can be accomplished through e-mail newsletters with sample scenarios or through a written annual commitment, in which all staff sign an agreement to use appropriate communication. Have the medical staff sign one, have it enlarged, and display it over the visitor entry.

3. Leadership must demonstrate commitment to this process through their actions

They can do so in many ways, such as by ensuring not only that collaborative committees meet but also that participants are comfortable sharing their thoughts and concerns. Rapid response to disruptive behaviors is another example of leadership expressing their seriousness about it.

4. Recognize that doctors and nurses have learned to communicate in different styles and methods

Between 1995 and 2003, the primary cause of sentinel events was problems with communication, according to the JCAHO.[2] Nurses are taught to gather data, relay it verbally to the doctor, and include every detail in documentation. Physicians are taught to discover the problem and work out what needs to be done to fix it. How can you reconcile these methods of communication? Start with making staff aware of the differences.

5. Involve the staff-level nurse in teams and committees

Typically, as the manager, you are not in your department on a regular basis in the early hours of the morning. To measure patient and staff needs around the clock, however, we need to involve the people who are working during those times. Therefore, do not discourage nursing involvement by only holding meetings during the day—night shift staff need to sleep during the day. Instead, vary meeting and committee times to give off-shift staff an opportunity to participate actively. Some medical staff hold their meetings either very early in the morning or in the evening, and there is no reason nursing cannot do the same.

6. Identify success elsewhere and mimic it

Find elsewhere the success you are seeking, study how it was accomplished, and then model your organization's method on it. In building collaborative practices, our best resources are ourselves—we must share our successes with one another. Magnet facilities are great examples for us in this way as well, and any time spent on a field trip to see them in action is well worth it.

7. Relate patient outcomes to collaborative initiatives

It is one thing to feel a part of the process; it is another to actually see and work with the patient benefits related to it. Communicate data related to initiatives that involve collaborative practice agendas, and then educate staff as to how this information translates into improved patient care.

8. Building relationships requires patience

Be patient with yourself, your staff, and the overall organization as you identify goals and work toward attaining them. Changing and improving the practice environment by incorporating more teamwork and cooperation across departments and amongst professionals takes time. It will be an ongoing and continuous effort that does not have an end point. It is one of those projects that should not have a completion target date—if it ends, then you lose an important motivator for nurses to stay with the organization.

The benefits of participating in collaborative systems that improve patient care

How many times have you heard staff nurses talk about wanting to be more empowered to do things differently? Yet sometimes when we ask for input or involvement, there is a rush for the door because no one wants to participate. Managers and leadership need to realize that what they see as active involvement may not be what staff see.

Nurses who feel they are actively involved in patient care processes and decisions are more satisfied with their jobs. Your challenge is to explore more ways for nurses to feel empowered and involved, but you first have to step back and learn what their perceptions really are. You can do so through informal discussions in small groups, at staff meetings, or through written surveys. Some key questions to consider are as follows:

- If you could be empowered to do one thing around here, what would it be?

- Do you feel you need a policy or procedure in writing to validate all the things you are already empowered to do?

- What would motivate you to become more involved in patient issues related to your department?

- What is going on now in your environment that has turned you away from any desire to become more involved?

- Do you feel you are working in an environment where you can share your thoughts, concerns, ideas, or suggestions comfortably?

The responses to these questions will help you identify your next steps to motivate and encourage nursing involvement.

People need to see results

All too often, staff go to meetings, collect data, and talk about issues but never see any results. Thus, for staff to feel involved, follow-through is imperative.

Shared governance has become popular with nurses because it allows them to contribute to decisions about issues and processes and then actually see the results of their involvement. For example, try changing clinical medical staff committees into joint practice committees with both nursing and physician presence.

Daily collaboration

It's important to realize and appreciate that collaboration can occur spontaneously.[3] As leaders, we must point out to medical and nursing staff all the collaborative efforts that are in place every day.

Case study: Seamless teamwork

An elderly man is about to be discharged with the walker he brought to the hospital. The nurse notices the patient cannot ambulate safely with this walker and is concerned that he may fall. The nurse brings this issue to the attention of the physician, and together they discuss the options they could consider. The nurse calls physical therapy for their perspective, and a plan is developed for the patient to use a walker on wheels. The plan is brought to the physician, who agrees, and the patient is discharged with a new set of wheels. Although this situation may sound like basic nursing, it is a great example of interdisciplinary practice with collaborative effort between nursing, medical staff, and physical therapy.

Case study: Spontaneous teamwork

The ICU nurse manager is walking down the hallway and sees a surgeon. They exchange greetings, and the nurse manager asks the surgeon if she has a minute to talk while she walks with her. The nurse manager shares a concern about a new postop standard that affects ICU patients and relates it to a patient in ICU yesterday. The surgeon agrees that this issue is a concern. She mentions that there is a patient medication safety committee meeting that day and invites the nurse manager to attend and share her concerns and ideas for how to prevent the situation from occurring again.

Overcoming emotions

Collaboration is about relationships and therefore will involve emotions. At times, these emotions can become obstacles to the effectiveness of your efforts, which reminds us why objectivity is necessary to guide the changes in how physicians and nurses communicate, how patient care decisions are made, and how all employees are held accountable for disruptive behaviors. Consider professional burnout, differences on opinion from cultural perspectives, and the lack of negotiating skill many staff may have. Identify leadership who are charged not only with the physical energy to lead change but the emotional energy and integrity to do so.

References

1. Connie Linck, RN, CNAA, BC, MSN, and Susan Phillips RN, C, MSN, "Fight or Flight? Disruptive Behavior in Medical/Surgical Services," *Nursing Management* (May 2005). 47–50.

2. *Competency Manager Advisor,* HCPro, Inc. (February 2005), 7.

3. Deborah B. Gardner, PhD, RN, CS, Ten Lessons in Collaboration, *www.nursingworld.org,* January 2005.

Chapter 8

PROFESSIONAL DEVELOPMENT

Learning objectives

After reading this chapter, the participant should be able to

- identify education and training resources related to professional development
- discuss how a commitment to professional development aids recruitment and retention

More than money

Studies remind us about the important role salary plays in recruitment and retention, but they also identify other important reasons why people accept or remain at a job. One of the items that always makes the list relates to professional development. It might be stated as training, education, or ongoing development, but regardless of what you call it, nurses want training and, for the most part, truly enjoy continuing education programs that meet their learning needs. They also want to be treated and respected as professionals and sometimes find themselves trapped between what they learn professionalism is versus what they think it should be.

What is professionalism?

Demonstrating professionalism

As in any situation, the manager needs to set an example of professionalism, and when it comes to professional development, staff will watch to see what you do for your own personal training and growth. They watch what you wear and how you carry and present yourself with patients, medical staff, and with administration.

Lead by example

Demonstrate your own professionalism:

- At meetings or in other communications, reference something you learned from a class, self study CD, or article you read. Let staff know where the information came from.

"I was impressed by what I learned about verbally de-escalating angry patients and families in one of the sessions I attended at my conference last month. I brought copies of the handout material to our meeting today so I could share this information with you to get your insights to see whether it is an approach we should consider for our department."

- Post notices or place a note via e-mail or in the communication book when you are going to be away at a class.

"I will be out of town with my pager off during class time while I attend the update on changes in our state nurse practice act. When I return, I will fill you in on what is being proposed. In the interim, check this Web site for more details:"

- Attend some classes with your staff, such as an ACLS renewal course.

- Leave a copy of the brochure of a conference you will be attending, with the specific workshops you are scheduled for highlighted so staff can review them.

- If you are going back to college to obtain a degree, talk about your course, the professors, and what you are learning. Consider posting a countdown calendar for staff to see where you are in the program and what your timeline and goals are for completion.

- Demonstrate the importance of supporting your specialty organization by displaying posters, wearing a membership pin, or getting involved in state chapter efforts.

- Bring in your professional nursing journal issues to share with staff.

- Always follow the dress code policy. Look in the mirror before you leave for work, and ask yourself whether the patients and medical staff see from your physical appearance that you are an authority figure—and a professional one at that.

As you work toward implementing these practices, be careful not to set unrealistic expectations of the staff. They will not all run out and join their professional organizations, nor will they all read the conference brochure you posted, but they will all know that their manager is using current knowledge and skills to lead the patient care in their department. You are sending a strong message of professionalism, maturity, and accountability. These three elements related to professional development truly reflect its meaning and help us understand the enticing role it plays in nursing recruitment and retention.

1. Professionalism

What does this word mean to you as the manager, and what does it mean to your staff and the prospective staff you interview? It can imply many things, such as being an expert or being trained/skilled in a specialty. It is your professionalism that is reflected when you elect to show up for work wearing clean white shoes, instead of the same sneakers you wore when you mowed the lawn. Relate your personal definition of professionalism to that of your staff.

The manager can gain this insight by talking with staff and having them share amongst themselves their perceptions. Using group techniques, you can collect and share this information as part of a learning process at a staff meeting. Ask each nurse to write on a card two words or statements that define professionalism for them. Collect the cards and, using a grease board or flip chart, ask a staff member to read each response while another staff member writes them down for all to see. Refer to Figure 8.1 for a sample chart. While staff are writing down their comments, advise them that you have already written your definition of being professional and that you will share it with them after their cards are read and posted. Give staff an opportunity to discuss the responses from their peers, and then reveal your perception of being professional, which may look similar to Figure 8.2.

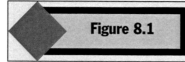

Figure 8.1	**Being professional is . . .**

Being skilled at what you do	////
Presenting yourself in an ethical manner	//
Having current knowledge in your specialty	///////
Acting with respect toward your coworkers and patients	//
Meeting the standards of what is expected of you	
Complying with rules and regulations of your profession	///
Working together as a team	

/ = for each person with a similar or like response

Figure 8.2	**The manager's perception of being professional**

Meeting the standards of your specialty

Behaving, dressing, and presenting yourself in an ethical and appropriate manner

Taking personal accountability for showing up at educational events, staff meetings, etc.

Maintaining a current knowledge base of your specialty

Supporting your specialty organization

In the next exercise, ask staff to write down one incident that has happened that they feel did not represent professional actions—and be careful to ensure that no one uses any names. Once again, collect and post these results, and open the floor for discussion. Doing so gives you and staff an opportunity to discuss actual scenarios that you or they would not want to represent your profession. Below are examples that could be discussed:

• A COPD patient entered the facility for a lab appointment through the wrong door and was met by a nurse taking a smoke break near the ED entrance.

- A nurse asks you to take care of a med order for her because she missed the last two update classes and doesn't know how to administer it. She is whining and complaining about all the required education the facility has.

No one wants to work in an environment where these types of behaviors occur on a regular basis. Nurses want to be surrounded by others who believe professionalism is important.

2. Maturity

How many times have you said to yourself, I just wish some of these people would grow up? Some nursing staff are having similar thoughts about some of their coworkers. They want to be part of a team where maturity sets the pace for character and decision-making. And as your staffing needs grow, you may find yourself in a position where you are accepting more new graduate nurses who are in their very first situation where they have to deal with work responsibilities, let alone nursing responsibilities.

Making decisions about when to take a lunch break can seem minimal in how they affect others, yet in nursing, such decisions may affect patient safety. It takes time and patience to help our new graduates grow and mature, and they deserve to receive help in the form of our demonstration of seasoned decisions and solid character that defines what being a professional is all about.

3. Accountability

Whatever you do, don't let staff know that accountability and empowerment are the same thing—because if you do, many of them won't want to be empowered any more. As managers, we hold ourselves accountable to ourselves, staff, patients, and the organization.

The professional staff nurse will want to be held accountable in the same manner and will be willing to do what it takes to show this level of responsibility. However, because there will always be staff who feel that they do not have to be accountable to anyone except themselves, management must step forward and be the entity holding everyone to the same level of accountability.

Case study: Accountability

Mary received a letter from the board of nursing stating that they had not received her renewal and that her license was due to expire that week. She realized that when she moved to a new apartment, she had neglected to send them her forwarding address. She took responsibility for this oversight, and she made time to drive the two hours to the office and pay the late fee to renew her license.

Michael is in the same situation, but he feels that the hospital should have a process in place to remind him. After all, he is busy with other things in his life. Are you going to hold Michael accountable? Will he be taken off duty without pay as soon as his license is invalid? Your staff are watching to see what will be done and are proud when the organization takes steps to ensure that nurses hold themselves accountable to such issues related to professionalism.

Case study: Attending classes

Jennifer had the same opportunities as the rest of the staff to select from one of four dates to attend a mandatory update educational session for the department. She did not attend any of them and did not let her manager know about any problems keeping her from doing so. The hospital's policy states that staff who do not attend cannot be placed on the time sheet without approval of the nurse manager. The night shift is short-staffed and Jennifer knows this, so she has signed up for her three twelve-hour shifts. Are you going to take her off the schedule? Once again, staff are watching you to see whether you will hold everyone accountable to the same level of responsibilities.

Your state board of nursing has enacted new standards regarding continuing education requirements, and you have posted some information, along with a Web site, for staff to use to reference the specifics. Stephanie is now in your office saying that she is angry that "you did not notify her" of these changes. She was unable to renew her license because she did not have adequate continuing education validation to present with her renewal application. Are you going to put the accountability back in her lap?

Here's a sample script for how you could respond to Stephanie: "Stephanie, if you look at your nursing license, it has your name on it—not mine, and not the hospital's. That means that you are personally accountable and responsible not only for knowing what the requirements are but for meeting them as well. It is unfortunate that you did not review the communication board two months ago when I posted the notice regarding this change."

Each time the manager takes steps to hold nursing staff accountable, they send important messages about professionalism. Staff who are accountable and responsible will walk with heads held high, knowing that you respect their choices and that you see them as the professionals they are.

Requirements for professional development

The education and training aspect of professionalism is driven from a variety of directions. Specific requirements may be set through various entities, such as the JCAHO, your state board of nursing, hospital policy, specialty standards, or state statutes. It is also a self-driven force, as people strive for professional development for reasons of personal fulfillment and challenge.

Encouraging education and training

Developing your nursing staff requires coaching from you, especially for newly graduated nurses. Develop a resource list that staff can use to access information about the requirements to obtain education, as well as information on where they can find the resources.

Figure 8.3 is an example of a resource list for nurses who work in an emergency department. Fulfilling the training and educational needs of nurses should be viewed from both a short-

| Figure 8.3 | Professional development resources |

Organizations
  Emergency Nurses Association
  American College of Emergency Physicians

Journals
  Journal of Emergency Nursing
  Annals of Emergency Medicine

Books
  Emergency Nursing Bible
  Standards of Emergency Nursing Practice
  Emergency Nursing Procedures

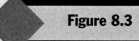

Figure 8.3   **Professional development resources (cont.)**

Web sites
> www.ena.org
> www.acep.org
> www.emedhome.com
> www.enw.org

Colleges
> State Community College for classes on
>> PALS, ACLS, BTLS, TNCC, ENPC

Other programs
> Life Flight Program has classes on
>> PALS, TNCC
> Critical care program
>> Emergency nursing basics

term and a long-term perspective. Nurses may need to acquire certain skills for the position they hold now, but it is important to incorporate education that gives them a focal point for some of their long-term goals, which may be three years from now.

Managers need not feel threatened by the nurse who is returning to school part time. Imagine a situation in which John, one of your nurses, is attending school part time to become a nurse practitioner. You may worry that you'll lose the best clinical night person you have when John finishes school, but you have to remember the bigger picture. John may be moving on to other opportunities when he completes his goals, but look at the benefit you, the staff, and the patients are gaining while he is there for two more years. For now, John is

- a role model and mentor for staff

- a nurse with advanced assessment skills who can help his peers improve their own assessment skills

- a staff member with a higher sense of responsibility, both clinically and ethically

- a nurse who, while still in training, will focus on identifying particular clinical concerns that will improve patient outcomes

Another way to approach the situation is from the professional development perspective by asking yourself whether there is a need in the department that can be filled by John when he completes his training. Have you been thinking of hiring a clinical nurse specialist or wound care nurse? Part of our jobs as managers is to help staff develop their professional growth by guiding them in career choices.

Highlight your staff's successes

John will always remember the manager who supported him while he was in school, and he will take particular pride in the organization that backed his decision with a flexible schedule. This is an amazing recruitment and retention opportunity and an example of where you can use your bragging rights to aid in recruitment and retention efforts. Shout John's successes from the rooftops by

- posting on the hospital Web site (with his permission) a photo of John with "his story," describing his career choice and how he is making it happen

- placing a photo of you and John in the local community newspaper when he completes his Nurse Practitioner program, and include comments about his career path and how the organization supported him

- using the same photos and stories in your nursing recruitment ads or brochures

You should be very proud of what John has accomplished and to be part of an organization that supports this type of professional development.

Offer access to continuing education

Encourage professional development by providing programs such as on-site education. Your time and financial investment in such programs will come right back to you in recruitment and retention—managers with reputations of supporting nursing education are the ones whose vacancies fill quickly. When staff are supported and encouraged to attend educational offerings, it sends a message that the organization values them and their capabilities.

Nurses feel appreciated when their organization goes a step further and sends them off-site to national conferences. When you look at the overall costs for doing so compared to the cost of recruiting and orienting another nurse, the numbers speak for themselves.

Your role in shaping future careers

Now that you realize that professional development is more than ensuring that staff renew their CPR cards, position yourself with information that helps you look at your staff's individual career choices and paths. Some will prefer to stay at their current level, but five years from now, that may change. You never know when the opportunity you give a nurse will affect the development of a peer. Using tools such as the ones in Figure 8.4 and Figure 8.5 can help both you and the new graduate nurse or experienced nurse plan for current and future skills and educational needs. Figure 8.6 can be customized to set long-term goals.

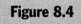

| **Figure 8.4** | Department of nursing—professional development |

New graduate nurse

Employee name

Date of hire

Date of graduation from nursing school

Date of successful completion of nursing boards

Education	Target date	Resource	Date completed/comments
Basic arrhythmia	After 90 day probation	In-house class	Next class June 14/15
Wound care update	30 days of hire	In-house CD/self study	Completed April 10 88% on written assessment tool
ACLS prep course	After 6 months of hire	Community college	Scheduled for fall class
Transitioning from student to professional	30 days of hire	In-house class	Completed—evaluation tool turned in

Figure 8.5	**Department of nursing—professional development**

Experienced nurse

Employee name

Date of hire

Department/specialty

Current certifications

Professional development plan for 2005–2006

Education	Target date	Resource	Date completed/comments
ACLS	Fall 2005	In-house training	
PALS	Feb 2006	Community college	
Charge nurse training	2005	In-house training	Completed March 2005 Performing charge position prn
Advanced EKG interpretation	2006	Off-site seminar	Registration application submitted
Excel basics	2005	In-house session	Signed up for class on Sept 8

Additional professional development:

1. Has requested on own time to spend a shift with one of our nurse anesthetists
   Scheduled for August 10

2. Presented a class for the middle school science teacher on "10 reasons not to smoke"

Notes:

This employee has expressed an interest in going back to school to become a nurse anesthetist.

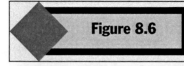

Figure 8.6	Professional development—career path

Today's date

Name

Current position

Department

	1 year	2 years	3 years	4 years	5 years	Comments
Charge nurse						
Supervisor						
Returning to school						FNP program
Changing to a different specialty						Labor and delivery
Advancing to a nursing management position						

At this time, I am professionally content with my position and role

Tie professional development into recruitment and retention

As you continue to develop what you offer nursing staff in terms of their professional growth, always consider how you can tie these efforts into recruitment and retention:

- Place a photo and story in the local newspaper about the nurses who recently completed their specialty certifications

- Use your Web site to spotlight quotes from new grads and new hires about how wonderful your orientation process is and how they are elated with the ongoing education offered on-site at no cost

- Work with a community newspaper to have nurses involved in writing a monthly column related to a timely health issue

Employees want professional development

The Society for Human Resource Management addressed the issue of staff turnover in a survey that examined what people were really looking for in their jobs and careers. The second biggest reason that they would begin searching for a new job was dissatisfaction with potential career development. The third reason was readiness for a new experience. This information highlights the importance of your professional development efforts.

When focusing on the retention side of professional development, ask yourself these questions:
- What processes are in place to have staff provide some of the training themselves?

- What opportunities are there for staff to cross-train so they can decide whether they want to pursue other specialties or interests in the organization?

- When was the last time you gave staff an opportunity to express what their other interests are and how they see themselves incorporating them into their job?

- How often are staff given an opportunity to participate in committees or teams?

- Are staff able to use some of their talents, skills, and knowledge at occasions outside the building, such as at a health fair or a senior citizen blood pressure screening?

Case study: Focusing on what really matters

Kevin is about to graduate nursing school. He has worked as a nursing assistant for a year, and he knows that this exposure has increased his comfort level when working with patients. As he excitedly starts setting up job interviews, he is overwhelmed by all the offers for hourly salary rates, sign-on bonuses, and other tempting incentives. However, many of the nurses he worked with previously had given him advice about what to look for in his first job, and they suggested that he focus on what the organizations offered in terms of orientation and ongoing education.

After all those years of working for little more than minimum wage, Kevin is initially drawn by the glitter of the salary. However, those experienced nurses had a great effect on him, and he eventually opts for a lower-paying job that has an excellent program for new graduate orientation and a department manager who is overtly committed to ongoing training for the staff. As he settles into his new role, he hears feedback from his former schoolmates and realizes that he has made the best decision for his professional development. His schoolmates share stories of their experiences, ranging from one who receives little new graduate support to one who is expected to start as a charge nurse on the night shift in the next month and who is so overwhelmed by this responsibility that he is looking for a new job already.

Professional development should begin from day one of graduation and be an ongoing process throughout a nurse's career. Our new graduates need some dedicated time and guidance to transition in their roles. Facilities with these programs are more enticing to the new graduate nurse.

Kaye and Jordan Evans write that, "Our research shows that more than any other single factor, people stay in an organization because of opportunities to stretch, grow and learn."[1] Relating this research to professionalism is vital to reducing employee turnover and hiring the best for the team.

Use the pyramid (see Figure 8.7) as your guide that ties all this together. From the time that you make a decision to hire or recruit an individual nurse, think about how you will encourage him or her relating to career goals, education, and training. Your leadership will drive his or her professional development and, therefore, the standards of the department.

Quality patient care will result from your staff's professional development, and patients will see their caregivers' commitment to delivering the very best. Staff feel good about being part of a team they know is qualified and competent to meet the needs of their patients. Never forget the importance of your role as you recruit, interview, and work to keep the wonderful nurses you already have.

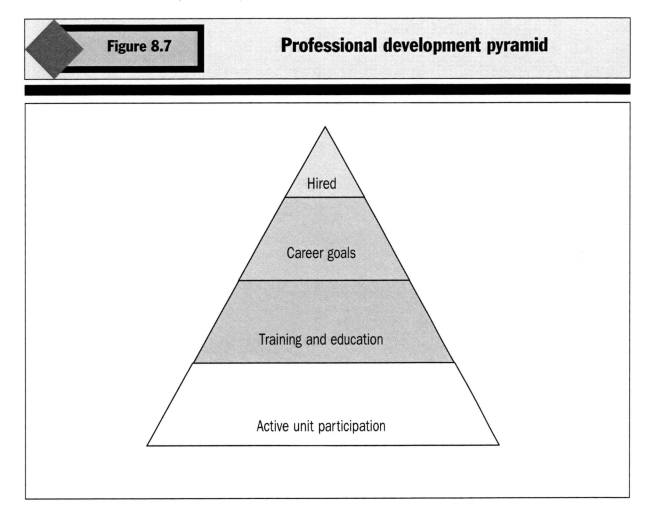

Figure 8.7 — **Professional development pyramid**

References

1. Kaye and Jordan Evans, *Love 'Em or Lose 'Em,* San Francisco: Berrett-Koehler Publishers, 1999.

Chapter 9

RECOGNITION AND REWARD PROGRAMS THAT PROMOTE RETENTION

Learning objectives

After reading this chapter, the participant should be able to
- identify ways to reward staff for exceptional performance
- list essential aspects of the performance review that enhance retention

The importance of recognition and reward programs

Recognizing and rewarding employees are integral components of any retention program. Work in healthcare organizations is laborious and stressful, and most nurses choose their career because of an inherent desire to make a difference in people's lives. Recognition of their contributions to quality patient care and peer relations affirms that they are succeeding in making a positive difference.

Most healthcare employees are motivated by a passion for caring for others—both patients and colleagues. For a majority of nurses, recognition and reward for exceptional contributions to patients and colleagues demonstrates appreciation, value, and caring by peers, managers, administration, and the healthcare organization.

Principles of recognition and reward

Consider several principles as you develop recognition and reward programs and activities. There's nothing worse than thinking you have a thoughtful, exciting new way to recognize staff only to realize that your employees did not appreciate the effort at all.

Be genuine in all of your activities, and make recognition personal

You must be sincere and genuine in any recognition or reward action. Staff members quickly realize if your words or actions are appropriate for the occasion. Your thoughts do not have to be inspired, but they must be inspiring. It can be as simple as, "I appreciate what you do," or, "You are an important part of our healthcare team." Keep thank you notes available at all times, and make a goal of writing at least five every few weeks. Keep them simple and personal. Most people have experience working with a supervisor who only provides a pat on the back and positive comments when he or she wants you to work an extra shift—as she begins to commend you on your work, you're already thinking of reasons why you can't work on the weekend. The purpose of recognition and rewards are to sincerely thank someone for something already given, not to warm them up for something you want.

Award recognition and rewards fairly and equitably

A cardinal rule of healthcare is to "do no harm," and the same holds true for recognition and rewards. Your goal is to demonstrate appreciation for a job well done, but you don't want to alienate certain groups of employees. For example, although it's great to recognize nurses during Nurses Week, you'll want to make sure you have an opportunity to recognize respiratory technicians, physicians, and housekeeping staff as well. Make sure you have a fair and equitable process for selecting recipients. Develop criteria for each award that is given. If you serve as the master of ceremonies for an award event, never say, "the winner is . . . " but rather, "the award goes to . . . " Also, describe the specific behavior that was observed and that warranted the recipient receiving the award.

Ask staff how they would like to be recognized

You might form a Recognition and Reward Task Force to survey or hold a brainstorming session to determine ways staff members prefer to be recognized.

Case study: Inappropriate recognition

Maria was a quiet, reserved nurse who had performed excellent care for several years and was rewarded with an Excellent Patient Care Award. As she received the award in front of the group, she was asked to say a few words. It was immediately obvious that she had no idea she would be asked to speak and was surprised and embarrassed in front of the group.

Some people prefer death to speaking in front of a group, so always ask staff whether they would like a few moments to speak. If you plan to do a bulletin board and include staff photos, ask them how they feel about it. Some staff prefer no public recognition, but they may really like to be recognized in a private manner, such as with a letter or a certificate. Others love to be recognized publicly. Therefore, know which staff prefer which types of recognition.

Individualize recognition activities

Know your employee's life interests and priorities, and look for a great recognition or reward action that matches those interests. If an employee is an avid golfer, their reward might be a dozen of their favorite golf balls or a round of golf at a local course. For someone who knits or crochets, it might be the latest wool, or scarf pattern. The most effective actions match the employee's life interests and priorities.

Case study: Personal touch

Rhonda was a nurse recruiter who consistently exceeded recruitment goals and was being recognized for the fourth year in a row for her exceptional recruiting. The director of the human resources department asked her to attend the annual awards luncheon to accept the beautiful plaque the hospital usually provided. As the director delivered the award, Rhonda remarked, "Thank you, but to be honest, I have a wall full of these awards."

Rhonda continued to excel, and in year five, she once again won the award. The director had learned an important lesson, and she knew the love of Rhonda's life was her three year-old Cocker Spaniel named Samantha. She secretly arranged for a colleague who kept Samantha when Rhonda was out of town to bring her to a professional photographer to have photos taken. At the luncheon, as Rhonda walked to the front, the director said, "We hope you know how much we love what you do for us," as she unveiled the beautiful framed photo of Samantha. Tears flowed from Rhonda's eyes, and for the first time in a long time, she was speechless.

Make recognition and reward a part of your work culture

Make formal and informal recognition and reward a usual and customary part of your every day work life. Establish formal recognition programs such as Employee of the Month and Employee of the Year. Encourage staff to recognize positive behaviors in colleagues on a daily basis. Make recognition a part of your staff meetings.

Make formal recognition events thoughtful and majestic

If you already have a nice Employee of the Month or Employee of the Year event and have held it for several years, you must make the event fresh and engaging each year. You do not need to increase your cost for the event, but you do need to integrate new thoughts and ideas. For example, change the theme or change table decorations. You must romance your staff: The ceremony must be thoughtful, it must be meaningful, and it must include something unexpected.

Even though you provide an excellent luncheon and special memento to celebrate Nurses Week, it won't be long before attendees begin to say, "It's the same thing we've been doing for the past three years." Mix it up. You might do a casual luncheon one year and a dress-up dinner the next. When recognizing employees of the year, you might use an "Evening of Stars" theme. One recruiter used an Oscar night theme and hired an actor who performed as a live Oscar statue.

Examples from practice

Golden Bethune, Director of Nursing at Centra Health in Lynchburg, VA, has a deep commitment to retaining staff, and efforts for employee recognition and reward play a central role in creating an engaging workplace. Centra Health employs the following examples of formal and informal recognition and reward activities and peer recognition activities, and these proven practices can be adapted for any organization.

Formal recognition and rewards

Create a formal recognition committee to nominate and submit applications to recognize staff. Committee membership consists of nurses who represent all service lines and nursing units. Staff are chosen for unit- and hospital-wide recognitions. The committee also submits applications for state and national recognition programs for nurses:

- Provide a recognition breakfast, lunch, and dinner for nursing assistants and licensed practical nurses who work to advance their skills to higher certification or license levels.

- Recognize staff who have perfect attendance on a quarterly basis.

- Award a quarterly unit "Spirit Award," and make each recipient eligible for an annual "Spirit" prize. Awardees names are placed into a drawing for a vacation trip, conference attendance fees, or some other meaningful prize.

- Develop and display an Employee of the Month bulletin board.

- Hand out "Staff Awards" at each staff meeting. Throughout the month, have staff e-mail the manager about something great a coworker has done. At the end of the staff meeting, recognize staff members and give a small gift and a certificate of appreciation.

Informal recognition and rewards

- Recognize a staff member for a job well done in front of other staff on a daily basis.

- Hand out movie tickets for two when someone needs encouragement, and include a note that says "Look at the big picture and know you are appreciated."

- Display banners that list the years of service for all staff. Provide a tally to demonstrate the total years of service on a unit.

- Forward to the entire staff e-mails you receive that name a specific person for some accomplishment, and ask them to join you in congratulating that team member. Provide a token gift.

• Begin each staff meeting with recognition of staff members mentioned on patient satisfaction surveys or thank you cards from patients.

• Develop an "Extra Mile Award" for extraordinary accomplishments outside your staff's normal jobs.

• Create a "pass along award." It may be some sort of trophy or stuffed animal that has meaning to the group. For example, you might establish the "Stuffed Monkey" Award to recognize quality performance with a theme of "No Monkey Business Here." Establish a rule that the recipient must pass the award along to another deserving person within two weeks of receiving it.

• Give individual staff members their own day. Recognize special people, achievements, or actions by declaring a work date as their day. Announce that next Tuesday is "Chris Smith Day," and ask all the staff to say or do something to contribute to the celebration.

• Recognize good performers by addressing the problems of poor performers. Letting others get away with sub-par behavior is a slap in the face to the majority of those who carry their share of the load—and more.

• Frequently point out what a great team you have.

• Send pizza with a "thanks for all you do" note when things are hectic on a unit.

• Buy fruit or candy, and place them around the unit with thank you notes.

Encourage peer recognition

• Place a journal on each unit, and dedicate it to the staff at the beginning of the year for them to write when coworkers do something nice or above and beyond expectations, so they can share each other's accomplishments.

- Encourage staff to e-mail you with good things about each other, and read the notes in staff meetings.

- Develop recognition stickers and make them available for staff to give each other when they do something good. For example, a sticker might read, "I made a difference today!"

- Encourage staff to provide a verbal thank you to coworkers on a daily basis.

- Put up a monthly "Caught Ya" bulletin board. Place colorful sticky note pads on each unit, and ask staff to write things about each other when they catch them doing something good above and beyond their normal job requirements. During February, use sticky notes in the shape of hearts.

- Supply a "recognition box" with cards, sticky notes, happy-face stickers, and other supplies, and place it in a common area. Encourage people to use material from the box frequently to acknowledge coworkers' good performance. Remember that you set the example.

A pat on the back or acknowledgement provides positive reinforcement. In the busy, hectic, stressful days of providing quality healthcare, it can reaffirm that they are making a difference in peoples' lives. Make recognition and rewards a part of your everyday work culture. Make it genuine. Make it personal. Make it meaningful.

Performance reviews are vital to retention

Case study: A waste of time?

Amanda has been a critical care nurse at her facility for eight years, and her annual review is coming up next week. The evaluation process at her facility offers no challenges for a nurse with Amanda's experience, and she views it as a waste of her time. A different perspective is provided by her boyfriend, Zack, who has been an OR nurse for five years at a different hospital. Since Zack's new OR manager, Sandra, started two years ago, employees have actually become excited about preparing for their annual reviews, and turnover has decreased.

Why performance reviews matter

Amanda's lack of an effective performance review may contribute to her lack of commitment toward her manager and her facility. If employees are not committed, they're likely to look for more attractive options elsewhere. This is one reason why effective performance reviews are vital retention tools that should become part of your ongoing retention efforts.

To better understand the importance of the relationship between performance review and staff retention, consider the above scenarios. What is Zack's manager doing that has her staff viewing their annual reviews positively? Reflect for a few minutes on comments often heard from nurses when asked about performance reviews or annual evaluations:

- "The only purpose of my annual review is to determine what percentage salary increase I get. For me, the 2.5% difference isn't worth the time of the review."

- "What performance are they reviewing? Everyone knows it doesn't matter how many inservices you skip or how rude you are—those people are still here, aren't they?"

Amanda may still be at her job despite her attitude about the annual review, but the important question is whether her performance is up to par. You can hang onto all the employees you want, but if they are poor performers, would you want to be a part of that team?

Evaluate your programs

An effective retention program needs to incorporate performance reviews that accomplish something and that both management and staff can trust. Before you begin a program or revitalize your existing one, consider that an effective program should clearly identify employees' strengths and weaknesses and guide them in goal setting. It also should support the manager's efforts.

Keep ongoing records

Think back to your experiences as a new manager, when you reviewed previous evaluations of staff. It's likely that, as you were reading some of them, you were thinking, "Someone must have put the wrong name on this one because there is no way that Kevin does all these things. I may have only been here three months, but I know he is rarely on time." Remember these enlightening moments the next time you are unsure of whether to document something on an employee's annual review. The process is not just for the employee—it is also for the manager, the organization, and any new manager that may step into that role unexpectedly.

Four steps to effective performance reviews

Follow these steps when reviewing how you currently work with staff at the time of their annual review or evaluation.

1. Setting the stage

Helping the employee feel prepared is as important as getting yourself ready, and you can accomplish this goal in numerous ways.

For example, send a letter or e-mail to employees that confirms the date and time of the review. Outline any material they are required to bring with them. Ask them to review a copy of their job description, and plan to discuss it. Remind them about where they can find this (such as in the department policy manual; do not include a copy of it with the letter). You may consider having them present five charts that demonstrate evidence of documentation standards or, possibly, a list of the continuing education activities in which they have participated during the past year.

Encourage them to bring copies of letters from coworkers or patients that recognize their efforts as a way to demonstrate the importance of their role to the department and the organization. Because coaching the employee to set goals is such an important aspect of this annual review, take the opportunity in your letter to include a worksheet to help guide them in setting these goals. (See Figure 9.1).

2. Manager preparations

Remember, the annual review should not be the first time employees hear negative or positive comments regarding their performance. They should be able to walk in to the meeting with no surprises thrown at them. You should be prepared with the following:

- Documentation to support your discussion of both positive and negative comments. Include copies of letters or notes from their peer group, evidence of time sheets with tardy dates if attendance is an issue, or incident reports from multiple occurrences of similar events.

- A clear perspective on what you want to communicate about their work performance.

- How you see them getting more involved in patient outcomes.

- A plan that includes clear expectations and timelines for changes in unacceptable behavior.

- Resource tools to validate your comments or plan of action (See Figure 9.2).

Figure 9.1	Goals worksheet

Name: _____

Job title: _____

Today's date: _____

Short-term goals

Professional:

In the next year, I would like to do the following:

Add _____ to my job description

Take _____ continuing education classes

Work on projects related to improving _____

Long-term goals

In the next 3–5 years I would like to do the following:

Have completed _____

Make these changes in my job _____

Have accomplished _____

Obtain certification in _____

| Figure 9.2 | **Manager resources for the annual review process** |

- Employee/hospital handbook

- Mission/Vision statement

- Department goals

- Applicable written policy or procedure

- Employee's current job description

- Previous year's evaluation for comparison and reference

- Copies of any regulations being discussed from JCAHO, OSHA, etc.

- Attendance records related to shifts, staff meetings, etc.

- Copies of patient charts that express good documentation skills

- Emails or letters complimenting the employee

- Records of committee involvement

- Salary history/information

Source: Shelley Cohen et al., Core Skills for Nurse Managers: A Training Toolkit. (Marblehead, MA: HCPro, Inc., 2004), 163–164.

Case study: Motivate

Brian: I don't care about the goals thing. Just put down that I'll renew my ACLS again: it's due this year for re-certification. Not everyone wants to go to Nurse Practitioner school, you know.

Manager: You are right about that—I have no aspirations to go to Nurse Practitioner school—but that doesn't mean I don't have any goals. For example, on my performance review, I put down that one of my goals was to take a health finance course to better understand the budget process. Setting goals isn't always about taking a class or achieving certification. It is about where you see yourself heading over the next year or two while you are in this job. So, with that in mind, where do you see yourself over the next year?

Brian: I do think about the time I am away from my kids and wish I could be there to do more things with them. I wish I wasn't gone so much—I miss lots of their school stuff that I wanted to be a part of now that they are a little older.

Manager: I appreciate your sharing that with me because it will help us set your goals for next year. You mentioned that you wanted more time for the kid's school activities, so have you thought about taking a six-month core position for weekends only that would give you Monday through Friday off? At the end of the six months you can decide whether you want to renew it or not. With the great feedback I get on your team leading skills, you would be perfect for shift charge status on weekends.

Brian: I didn't know you could stop the core status after six months. Can I sign up for that?

3. Focus on the goals

Goal setting has to be perceived by the employee as more than filling in the blanks on a form. If the manager minimizes the goals, the employee will never get the connection between job performance and having aspirations or ambition to do more.

This conversation has allowed the manager to identify the catalyst that will help Brian meet a personal need, which will thereby enhance his professional performance. At the same time, the manager may gain an effective leader for the weekend team. By working together to set goals, the manager sets out on a communication path to try to find what inspires and motivates the employee. Remember, employees who are happy and fulfilled with their home status reflect similar characteristics at work.

When employees know that their manager supports their goals and are asked to be a part of the solution for challenges in the department, then they become team players. This feeling leads to commitment, which is your retention motivator. The real test for the manager is to find a process that allows to you to incorporate the annual review into daily practice. Gather information throughout the year. Make small notes on staff performance, send e-mails to staff, talk to people at change of shift, and stop waiting for the annual performance review to be the one time when employees hear that they are doing a good job. Time spent with staff both on a formal and an informal basis provides both the employee and the manager with an opportunity to look at performance issues more frequently.

4. Have the employee feel a part of the change process for improvement

Prepare key questions that help prompt effective communication between the manager and the staff nurse. Consider providing the employee with this list of questions, along with the letter you send confirming his or her appointment for the review.

- If you had the power to change just one thing about this department, what would it be?

- Is there anything you have accomplished over the past year of which I am not aware that you would like to share with me?

- You are such an asset to this department and I appreciate all of your efforts and would like to know what motivates you to come to work every day?

- Where do you see our department heading in light of the recent issues and challenges we discussed at our last staff meeting?

- What can I, or our facility, do to help you do your job more effectively?[1]

The role of the senior nurse executive in recruitment and retention

A vast portion of the retention effort falls on the shoulder of the nurse manager. In today's world, mid-level managers are seeing their position shift to that of nurse recruitment/retention officer. Where does this leave the nurse executive in relation to this vital piece of patient care?

Without specific guidelines and goals, the senior nurse executive may be completely out of the loop until there is a crisis, such as a large turnover issue.

Become involved

To play an effective role in the recruitment and retention of nurses in your organization, consider these necessary functions of the nurse executive.

Leadership development: Ongoing leadership development for the mid-level manager is critical to the success you will have in retaining the nurse managers that work with you

Direct involvement: Become directly involved in various aspects of recruitment and retention. Have monthly data forwarded to you regarding turnover, overtime, agency staffing. Have exit interview forms from nurses copied for your review and follow-up. Discuss the recruitment and retention status of nursing at your regular manager meetings

Visibility: Make yourself visible to the new hires. Introduce yourself at nursing orientation. Once a month, meet with a newly hired nurse for coffee to get his or her perspective on the hiring process, orientation process, and job satisfaction.

Support: Support the orientation process. Allocate and support necessary funds for appropriate and productive orientation programs. Implement indicators for a quality review process of the orientation program. Have this data shared with all nurse managers and set goals for improvements.

Listen: Approach some of the seasoned nursing staff and ask them what keeps them there. Ask what they would like to see implemented by the organization to help retention efforts.

Nursing staff want to feel a connection to the chief nursing officer, partly for professional reasons, but also because they want you to know what a great job they are doing. Making time for them leaves a perception that you want to be aware of issues and that you really do believe that the nurse at the side of the patient is the most pivotal person in healthcare delivery. Go to a department where three nurses recently attained their specialty certifications, and have a picture taken with them for the newspaper or hospital Web site. Having pride in your profession not only provides a model for what we want to see in nursing staff but also leaves staff with a feeling of self-worth that motivates them to stay.

References

1. Shelley Cohen, et al., *Core Skills for Nurse Managers: A Training Toolkit* (Marblehead, MA: HCPro, Inc., 2004), 168.

Chapter 10

ESTABLISHING AN ACADEMIC PIPELINE

Learning objectives

After reading this chapter, participants should be able to

- identify methods to recruit young people into healthcare careers
- discuss the value of establishing relationships with schools of nursing

Creating nurse supply pipelines through academic partnerships

Schools of nursing and health professionals programs are the renewable sources of healthcare professionals you count on from year to year. Therefore, it's in the best interest of any healthcare organization to develop partnerships with these schools and programs to assist in student recruitment, student retention, faculty recruitment, faculty retention, clinical and classroom space, and even funding.

Recruit into the health professions

For many years, hospitals and healthcare employers have focused recruitment efforts only on schools of nursing, which cater to a group of people who have already decided to enter the healthcare profession. But if you focus on people before they reach that point, you can actively recruit people into the healthcare profession and expand your pool of potential employees.

Consider recruiting people into the health profession as a long-term strategy. Target youth, second-career individuals, older workers, and displaced workers. Provide opportunities for members of each of these groups to gain insight into the challenges and rewards of health-care careers. You might hold career fairs, volunteer programs, shadow programs, or even summer healthcare career camps.

High Point (NC) Regional Health System provides a "Promoting Advancement for Teens in Healthcare" (PATH) Program. The PATH Program is a student volunteer experience that selects sixty high school students to volunteer for fifty hours in the summer. The program is directed by hospital volunteer services, and each student gets to experience many aspects of care, as well as being required to attend classes on customer service, health and wellness, and healthcare careers.

Highlight the variety and potential of healthcare careers

People choose a career in nursing and healthcare because they want to "help people" or "make a difference in people's lives." Share your own story about how you, as a healthcare professional, have achieved positive patient outcomes. Develop a two-minute personal experience story that describes how a patient who was experiencing several healthcare challenges achieves a positive outcome.

Develop several such stories to use for different occasions. For example, have different ones to share with middle or high school students and another for second-career or displaced workers. For the latter groups, you could share a story of career growth and satisfaction, such as how an employee began working in housekeeping, and then through encouragement, financial assistance, and personal support is now working as a higher-level healthcare professional in your organization.

Young people have several misperceptions about nursing and healthcare careers. As you develop stories, materials, or presentations for youth, highlight the following areas to challenge their preconceptions and to illustrate how nursing is an interesting, challenging, and diverse career.

We need smart people in nursing

Nursing is an intellectually challenging career, but many youth do not think you need to be smart to become a nurse. The general perception is that nurses take orders from physicians and that it does not require an intelligent person to carry out physicians' orders. Therefore, when you talk with young people, let them know that nurses must keep up with the latest nursing knowledge and that learning will be a life-long endeavor.

We need decision-makers in nursing

Some young people believe that nurses are not autonomous professionals. Once again, the perception is that nurses only carry out physicians' orders. Therefore, talk with youth about how the nurse is a collaborative member of the healthcare team and is responsible and accountable for the delivery of quality nursing care. Help them understand that nurse managers are responsible for multi-million dollar budgets and that, many times, it's the nurse who recognizes that immediate interventions are required to prevent negative patient outcomes. Help them understand that nurses make decisions that affect patient outcomes each moment of the day.

There is a lifetime of variety in nursing

Most young people assume that all nurses work in hospitals. Although the majority does, let them know about the numerous other employment settings and environments, such as nursing homes, schools, rehabilitation centers, the military, cruise ships, or even with NASA astronauts.

Let them know that nurses work with a variety of patients, from newborns up to older adults. Also talk about the variety of specialties, including emergency room, orthopedics, critical care, pediatrics, dialysis, coronary care, psychiatry, rehabilitation, neonatal intensive care, and flight and transport. If you grow tired of working in one area, with some retooling and development of additional skills, you can transfer your skills to a different work setting or specialty.

Health careers offer opportunities for career progression

Many young people think that all you will ever do in nursing is bedside care. First, let them know that you can progress your career within direct care nursing. Many hospitals offer career advancement programs that allow you to advance in pay and responsibility based upon work experience, formal education, and certification. Talk about the roles of management, education, and research.

Nursing and healthcare is a role for both women and men

Young people and their parents continue to view nursing as a woman's work, but more and more often, both women and men choose nursing and healthcare careers. Both genders express an interest in helping people, and growing demand, increased wages, and few or no layoffs provide incentives to enter the field.

Avoid the squeamish factor

Although some youth are really into the "guts and glory" of healthcare, others state that they don't know if they can deal with giving an injection, looking at blood, or having a patient die while in their care. Be honest, but be sensitive if they ask questions about these areas.

Look at your organization's Web site

Most healthcare home pages focus on recruiting patients. Consider also placing a "Learn more about healthcare careers" button on your home page. If you have an "Employee of the Month" program, highlight the recipients, include photos, and describe their work responsibilities. Send an e-mail to local career exploration teachers in middle schools so they can explore your numerous careers. Include other activities that demonstrate the rewards and challenges of healthcare careers.

Practical strategies for educating young people about nursing and healthcare careers

Newspapers in Education

Most local newspapers provide the Newspapers in Education program. They contact teachers of career exploration courses and ask whether they would like to receive the paper at no charge to improve reading skills and to share career opportunities available in the local community. The newspaper then sells sponsorship space for career pages to local employers. Consider developing a page for this program on careers that you know will be in long-term demand. For example, you might do a full page that just generally focuses on nursing. Or if you feel that students need a better explanation of the different roles in nursing, you might sponsor a page each on nursing assistant, licensed practical nurse, registered nurse, and advanced practice nurse.

Speakers bureau

You may already have a speaker's bureau of healthcare professionals who provide health prevention education to the public. If you do, expand it to include employees who have stellar work experiences with your organization and are willing to improve their speaking skills. Include representatives from housekeeping, the business office, the human resources department, nursing, respiratory therapy, and so on. Develop a public speaking course to help them develop their success stories and to articulate to the public what they love about their careers. Look for opportunities to speak to community groups of youth, displaced workers, individuals considering second careers, and older workers.

Host or lead a youth group

Encourage some of your employees to host a youth group that is interested in learning more about healthcare careers. The YWCA and YMCA host several youth groups that focus on career exploration. Some communities have career explorer clubs, and both the Girl Scouts and Boy Scouts of America include badge and patch programs that focus on career exploration.

Coloring pages, puzzles, and textbook covers

Look for opportunities to increase youth awareness of healthcare careers. For example, you can develop and place coloring pages on your Web site that depict careers in your organization, then hold a coloring contest for Nurses Week or some other celebration.

Word puzzles focusing on medical terminology or healthcare careers are another strategy. You can place them on your Web site, or distribute them to your physicians for placement in their office waiting areas. Develop a variety of activities, and place your organization's logo on each one.

Encourage staff to get involved in community organizations

Most healthcare organizations encourage staff to provide community service, and often staff choose to be involved in health prevention, fundraisers, and other health-related activities. Educational systems play a major role in exposing youth to career choices, so encourage some of your staff to participate in the following roles:

- President or member of the Parent Teachers Association in an elementary or middle school
- Member of the local board of education for the public school system
- Member of a board of advisors for local private schools

- Health Occupations Students of America advisor or healthcare career advisor in a local high school
- Member of a school of nursing or allied health program advisory committee

Develop relationships with schools of nursing and allied health programs

Take a look at your recent new graduates, and analyze where they are coming from and the schools they attended. You may find that most of the programs are local, but you also may learn that you hire graduates from programs that are not in your immediate hiring region.

Make a list of the schools of nursing and allied health programs, and then determine where you have developed working relationships. Discuss with a recruiter or colleagues to make sure you have an organizational liaison that works closely with all of these programs to develop and maintain collaborative relationships. Designate someone in your agency to meet with the deans and directors at least once per year to discuss clinical rotations, student space needs, faculty orientation needs, and evaluations on student learning experiences. Some larger organizations are establishing full-time positions to work directly with the schools to arrange clinical rotations, faculty orientation, and so on.

Community meetings

Another strategy for coordinating student experiences and working together to address demand for healthcare professionals is to hold healthcare community meetings. For example, in Winston-Salem, NC, there is a Winston-Salem Healthcare Roundtable. The Chamber of Commerce hosts the meeting because it felt strongly that successful business and commerce depend upon the health and welfare of the area's citizens. Members of the Roundtable include local schools of nursing, hospitals, long-term care facilities, home health and hospice agencies, public school health occupations programs, and career awareness representatives.

Work with the schools

Develop working relationships with schools and educational programs by keeping faculty informed of what's going on in your facility. Send them copies of your organizational newsletter. Inform your staff about when and where student clinical experiences will be held.

Incorporate faculty into your workplace. Offer joint faculty-clinical appointments, or part-time employment opportunities. Use faculty to teach some of your continuing education programs. Use local faculty with research expertise to develop clinical research studies and opportunities.

Establish quality standards for great clinical experiences for your students. The nurse manager should welcome students in their first clinical conference, inquire about how the experience can be improved, and provide follow-up within a week. Emphasize your unit's commitment to providing quality care and a quality learning experience. Ask for input on how you and your staff can help with and improve their experience. Inform them on how you will implement their suggestions. Keep them up to date on your progress.

Establish relationships with students

It is important to develop relationships with nursing and allied health students before they graduate. Hold open houses and career fairs to share information about working in your organization and to begin developing relationships with the students. Visit schools, and provide pizza for student-sponsored events throughout the year. Advertise in college-related publications or student association magazines or newsletters. Host a senior reception two or three months prior to graduation. If you really want to make an impact, you might sponsor the pinning ceremony or pay for student pins.

Maintain data on each of these activities. You might do some type of gift give-away, which is an excellent opportunity to have students provide their names and addresses so you can begin to develop a mailing list. You could use your list to mail congratulation notes after graduation.

Ambassadors for your facility

The nurses already working at your facility make great ambassadors who can share their knowledge and provide real insight into your facility and working in healthcare.

Encourage your best nurses to give guest lectures at schools. You could offer a mentoring program in which nurses on your staff agree to serve as mentors for students in their final two years of their educational program. Make sure your preceptors are great ambassadors for your organization and that they provide challenging and rewarding student learning experiences.

When nursing students come to your facility for their senior clinical experiences, consider placing them on units where you will need nurses. In students' final semesters, many begin to see how their knowledge and skills actually contribute to positive patient outcomes. This is a real ego booster for them, and they really enjoy the patient and clinical experiences on those units.

Support the schools and students

Offer to help nursing and allied health programs improve student retention, as some programs lose more than 60% of their entering classes. More efficient programs provide more graduates, from which a larger number can be recruited by your organization.

Some schools require nursing assistant experience prior to entering a nursing program to make sure the student understands the realities of working in healthcare. Some hospitals provide the nursing assistant training for the students because it helps you develop a relationship with the student, provides needed nursing assistants, and gives the hospital a good look at the student's abilities and work ethic.

Another strategy you might consider is funding scholarships for nursing and allied health students. Scholarships are generally offered at $1,500–$2,000 per year and require a one-year work commitment per year of funding. They usually focus on junior or senior students.

Also consider developing an emergency fund for students in collaboration with local educational programs. Excellent students may be forced to drop out of a program because of small financial needs, such as an unplanned car repair bill. Therefore, establish an annual budget of $5,000, and tell faculty to let you know if emergency assistance is needed. Either mail or hand-deliver the check, along with a card that says, "We're investing in you because we think you'll make a great healthcare professional."

Incorporate students into your workplace, and develop stellar preceptor and mentor programs. Ask for volunteers for the programs, and use only those nurses who demonstrate strong interpersonal skills. Preceptors and mentors are ambassadors for your facility and can make or break possibilities of a future hire. Hire students as nursing assistants, and develop quality internship and externship programs. These programs give students an opportunity to learn about the realities of working with you, and it also gives you a chance to observe their work ethic and potential. Develop an orientation program, which can be individualized to transition the new graduate into the workplace.

Negotiate creative educational programs to increase capacity

Look for opportunities to expand your local healthcare professions programs. Negotiate to offer the following types of programs. Be prepared to provide financial and resource assistance to get these programs up and running.

Multiple graduations

Rather than offering entry in the fall and graduation in the spring, ask programs to consider continuous entry and graduation. Graduations occur in spring, summer, and fall, and you do not have to over hire in the spring to meet expected vacancies for the year.

Evening and weekend programs

There's a large cohort of second-career individuals who are interested in nursing and healthcare but who can't afford to stop work to attend school full time. Evening and weekend programs provide a workable option for those individuals to enter the healthcare work force.

On-site programs

Whether the programs are nursing assistant, LPN, RN, RN-to-BSN, MSN, or some other allied health program, having them on-site makes educational advancement more accessible to your current employees. Provide financial support and flexible scheduling options to encourage participation and success.

Online programs

Negotiate with programs to offer online academic programs and to help with clinical experiences. Staff can complete courses from the comfort of their homes. Consider installing a computer lab or developing a computer loan or subsidy program.

Accelerated programs

Accelerated programs meet the needs of second-career individuals who already have a bachelor's degree and are interested in becoming nurses. The program is completed usually in a twelve- to eighteen-month period. New nurses bring a variety of work experiences into the healthcare setting.

Paramedic-to-BSN programs

Paramedics can transfer credit hours from prior education to a nursing program. Paramedic-to-BSN programs usually attract a larger-than-normal proportion of men into the nursing profession.

Educational programs are your best renewable resource for healthcare professionals. Delivery of quality healthcare and services in your community requires close working relationships between both education and service-delivery organizations. Analyze your work force needs. Identify the resources each can contribute. Develop creative solutions, and negotiate win-win solutions and educational programs that meet the evolving healthcare and work force needs in your community.

Chapter 11

THE POWER OF METRICS

Learning objectives

After reading this chapter, participants should be able to

- identify the value of using metrics to measure recruitment and retention success
- list examples of recruitment and retention data that are useful to manage your work force

The power of metrics in recruitment and retention

More and more healthcare organizations are making work force development and planning an important part of organizational management. Traditionally, some employers have viewed nurses and other healthcare professionals as readily available commodities that can easily be purchased with sign-on bonuses, higher salaries, benefits, and other incentives as needed. With the current nursing shortage and consumer demands for quality care, employers are moving rapidly to conduct work force and workplace data collection and analysis systematically as an integral component for developing, retaining, and assuring a high quality healthcare work force and workplace.

Planning and ensuring that you have a quality healthcare work force and workplace are major challenges. Let's consider, for example, that a healthcare organization has 1,200 employees.

These employees are made up of a wide variety of healthcare professions, managers, and support personnel. Consider the different levels of educational preparation, ages, and cultural backgrounds. Each employee has her or his own thoughts, ideas, and motivators. Each brings different knowledge, skills, and expertise to the workplace. The individual human capital that each contributes can seem abstract until you identify methods for measuring it, and the same holds true for determining costs for turnover and being able to compare your success in recruiting and retaining staff. And consider the millions of processes that occur on a daily basis in an organization that provides healthcare. These things all can be measured and the results used for planning and improvements.

Making sense of metrics

The goal of metrics is to define it, measure it, and manage it. "It" can be whatever you'd like it to be. Workforce metrics are rapidly evolving as an integral component of managing a healthcare organization. The term "metrics" is becoming one of the buzzwords of the 21st century in work force development, and even consumers are beginning to ask, "What do your metrics look like?" Actually, they should be asking, "Which types of metrics are you using?" because there are so many different processes or outcomes you can measure. The possibilities are endless.

What is a metric?

A metric is a measurement of an activity, process, or other function. It involves data collection, analysis, and reporting, usually in a table or graphic format. Sometimes it's simply numbers or a prioritized list. Most often the data are quantitative and numerical in nature. Using metrics allows you to measure your organization's performance and progress over time or make a comparison to another unit, organization, or national or health system norm. Examples of human resource metrics recommended by the American Society of Hospital Human Resources Administrators include

- average net revenue per full-time equivalent (FTE)
- average net operating expense per FTE
- average compensation expense as a percentage of total operating expense
- average benefit expense per FTE
- average recruitment expense per hire
- vacancy rates

- retention rates
- turnover rates

As you can see, many of these metrics specifically demonstrate overall performance of the organization and the human resource department. You may want to consider factors and measurements that more specifically demonstrate performance with healthcare professionals, such as nurses or physical therapists with whom you work—or even the unit you work on, such as critical care or the operating room. Think critically about the types of data you need for daily decision-making. Effective use of workforce data can be a key tool to ensuring a quality staff and work place.

What to do with the data?

By analyzing metrics over time, you can establish benchmarks, or standardized measurements (usually averages) that allow you to compare your performance over time or against other units or healthcare organizations. Make sure when you're comparing your metrics to others that data are defined, collected, and analyzed in a similar manner. When comparing metrics, always make sure that you are comparing apples to apples, rather than apples to apricots: The first two letters of apples and apricots are the same, but the other letters are very different. The same can hold true for metrics—they can initially appear, sound, and look the same, but they may measure entirely different processes or outcomes.

Some managers use dashboards, which are collections of key performance indicators organized and presented in a format that is easy to read and review. Charts, graphs, and gauges are provided in a consistent format to assist strategic decision-making. Types of data that may be used to form one or more hospital dashboards include

- financial and funds management
- length of stay
- medication services
- mortality rates
- patient demographics
- patient satisfaction
- resource management
- total admissions
- unplanned returns to surgery

Each of these metrics can help the manager or administrator determine how the organization performs in the various areas and in what areas changes or corrections may be needed.

Work closely with human resources

Work closely with your human resources department as you consider developing metrics, benchmarks, or dashboards—you might be surprised at the data already being collected in your organization. With the use of computerized systems, much data is readily available. Be sure to collect data on a "need to know" rather than "nice to know" basis, and be very specific about what you need to make workforce and work place decisions.

Traditionally, human resources personnel have provided oversight of salaries and benefits, and other areas such as employee rights. Their roles are recently expanding to encompass strategic planning that includes the development of performance improvement measurements, and other work force metrics and benchmarks. Talk with individuals in your human resource department concerning metrics and benchmarks that will meet your work force planning needs. For instance, you may notice that you have many older nurses working on your unit and you'd like to determine the proportion that is within five years of the average retirement age. You may even need to pull nurse retirement records for the past five years to calculate the average retirement age for nurses for your hospital or unit.

Principles of human capital metrics

Hold discussions with your fellow managers or staff to consider which work force or workplace data you'll want to collect. Consider the following principles:

Never collect data for the sake of collecting data

There's always a cost involved in data collection, whether in time or in other resources. Even the time it takes for you to review the report is an important resource. Therefore, make sure you have a good rationale for how the information will help you in your decision-making process. Consider up front the amount of time needed to analyze data and turn it into useful information. Never collect data if it will not be analyzed.

Remember to measure processes, not people

Quantifying human capital in your organization is about measuring processes that occur or don't occur within your unit or organization. Consider measuring recruitment, hiring, orientation, learning, and retention processes. The goal is to identify what's working well and what improvements can make it work better.

Keep it flexible: Measure anything you want, anyway you want

When considering a purchase of blood pressure cuffs, you might be interested in determining the average number of times the piece of technology is actually used in a day to help you decide precisely how many to buy. You can certainly be flexible in how you take your measurements, but be aware that if you plan to observe for trends over time or you would like to compare your findings with other units or organizations, you'll need to define precisely what you're measuring and use the same measurement methods as those with whom you plan to compare your findings.

Measure consistently and use standard formulas

Using a standard formula and similar measurement processes allows you to make comparisons. If you measure your unit's vacancies in a unique manner that no one else uses, you cannot compare that figure with other organizations. Determine the type of data measurement you'll use. Most likely it will be quantitative, but you may find at times that qualitative data collection is your most appropriate method. Define your unit of measurement as one or more specific units or an entire organization. For example, is the vacancy rate you're discussing for the critical care unit, the medical surgical unit, or for your entire organization? You also may decide to provide certain metrics for specific groups, such as registered nurses, nurse managers, or cafeteria staff.

Also consider how often you'd like your measurements, such as weekly, monthly, or annually.

Make your metric simple

Don't make your metric more complicated than it has to be. Keep it simple. Define it, explain your measurement method, and be clear about what it does or does not include. For example, a colleague might ask you how many registered nurses work on your unit. Your first question is to establish whether he or she is interested in staff registered nurses or all registered nurses, since registered nurses work in the roles of manager, assistant manager, and so on.

Let's say the colleague wants to measure the number of staff registered nurses, but the assistant manager spends at least 80% of his or her time providing direct care—should that person be included? You can decide by defining staff registered nurses as those who spend at least 50% of their work time providing direct patient care.

Your next question might be whether he or she wants the total number of registered nurses working on the unit or the number of FTEs. FTEs would be based on the total hours worked on the unit, and because you have full-time and part-time positions, that number would be less than your total number of registered nurses. It can get pretty complicated. So if you only need to know the total number of registered nurses on your unit, keep it simple, and count the number of registered nurses' names on your work schedule.

Make sure you're measuring what you want to measure

Make sure you're measuring what you actually want to measure. Turnover data is a useful example. You might call it "Total Turnover" rather than "Turnover" if you're interested in the total number of employees who move from one position to another. Both "Voluntary Turnover" and "Involuntary Turnover" could make up "Total Turnover." Voluntary Turnover would include those employees who requested a position change or voluntarily terminated their position. Involuntary turnover includes employees for whom management mandated a position change or terminated their position. You may be interested in breaking your Total Turnover into "position changes" and "resignations and terminations." You can look at data in several different ways. Just make sure you're measuring what you want to measure.

Measure what's causing you the most pain

How do you know what to measure first? Determine what's causing the biggest issue among your staff. Use feedback from your employee satisfaction surveys, exit interview data, and performance appraisals. Maybe it seems to you that you're losing a large number of nurses on your evening shift, or maybe it seems to take forever to get new staff hired onto your unit. There's a world of things you can measure, but measure what's causing you the most pain and what is most likely to help you make decisions.

Healthcare work force and workplace metrics

As mentioned earlier, you do not need to measure every workplace process. Rather, identify the primary areas where you would like to improve and collect data that you feel will help you in the decision-making process. You may feel external pressure to have some metrics available to show information about your facility. The American Association of Colleges of Nursing recently recommended that new graduates request to review the following metrics before they accepted a position in a hospital:

- RN vacancy rate
- RN turnover rate
- Patient satisfaction scores (preferably percentile ranking)

- Employee satisfaction scores
- Average tenure of nursing staff
- Education mix of nursing staff
- Percentage of registry/travelers used

Practical examples of recruitment and retention data you can use to manage your work force

The following are some of the more common findings that are collected in hospitals and healthcare organizations on a regular basis.

Recruitment metrics

A number of measurements may be used to gauge recruitment success.

➤ **Number of open positions:** includes the total number of unfilled positions in an organization or on a unit.

➤ **Days to fill/hire:** this figure defines a day as 24 hours and is calculated from the date you post a position until the date the position is accepted.

➤ **Days to start:** this finding is computed from the date the position is posted until the date the new hire begins work.

➤ **Cost per hire:** this figure may only include advertising costs for a position. More recently, organizations are including orientation, decreased productivity, and other costs that are involved with fully incorporating new employees.

➤ **Number of hires by source:** usually identifies employees based on where they were prior to the hire. For example, it may be a hospital or it may be an educational program. Be clear about this figure, because it may also refer to how you're reaching your hires by advertising source. Did they learn about your openings by one of your newspaper or journal advertisements?

➤ **Net gain/loss per month:** includes the number of hires minus the number that exited your system.

Hiring process metrics

You may be interested in using a variety of metrics to improve your hiring process and even the quality of potential candidates you're attracting.

➤ **Number of applications:** total of completed applications you receive. You can tally them by position opening, but most often it is a total of all applications received on a monthly basis.

➤ **Application/interview ratio:** total number of interviews divided by the total number of completed applications received.

➤ **Interview/hire ratio:** total number of hires divided by the total number of interviews conducted.

➤ **Job offer declines by reason:** listing of rationale or comments concerning why a job offer is declined by a candidate.

➤ **Number of contract staff/contract labor hours:** number of contract staff used on unit or organization and total number of contract labor hours used.

Orientation process metrics

Organizations are realizing the importance of a quality orientation and data, which can help you rapidly integrate new employees into your work setting.

➤ **Competencies:** either through testing or a self-rated competency scale, employers identify skills and competencies of new hires. Competencies are based upon job descriptions and work responsibilities, and learning plans are created to develop individual competency needs.

➤ **Satisfaction:** includes feedback from new hires within the first month concerning how satisfied they are with the orientation process and work setting.

➤ **Length of orientation:** amount of time, usually in months and days, for the employee to work independently.

Retention metrics

Measurements pertaining to retention can help you determine areas that need immediate attention and also can help you with your long-term work force planning.

- ➤ **Vacancy rate:** usually vacancy rates include open positions divided by total positions on a unit or in an organization.

- ➤ **Turnover rates:** turnover rates usually include staff departures divided by total positions in a unit or an organization.

- ➤ **Percent of new hires:** percent of new hires is calculated by dividing the total number of new hires by the total number of employees. If you're calculating it for a unit, you use unit hires and unit employees. For the organization, you use total new hires and total employees.

- ➤ **Turnover rate of new hires:** calculated by dividing the number of new hires who depart by the total number of new hires.

- ➤ **Internal promotions:** includes the number of employees promoted from one role or position to another in your organization.

- ➤ **Number of terminations:** includes the number of employees that management or human resources terminates employment.

- ➤ **Average length of service:** dividing the sum of months worked by current employees by the total number of employees will provide the average months of employment of current employees.

- ➤ **Percent of employees eligible to retire without penalty:** calculated by dividing the number of employees who may retire with no penalty from your pension plan by the total number of employees.

- ➤ **Turnover rate of employees eligible to retire without penalty:** calculated by dividing the number of employees who actually do retire by the total number of employees.

Whether you're conducting work force planning, improving your recruitment and retention efforts, or building a case for increasing your recruitment and retention budget, metrics are powerful persuaders. Human capital may seem to be a challenge, but metrics provide the hard facts, numbers, and outcomes. Work force data collection, analysis, and review can help you ensure that you have a well-prepared healthcare work force, an exceptional work place, and quality patient care.

Chapter **12**

DOS AND DON'TS
OF RECRUITMENT

Learning objectives

After reading this chapter, participants should be able to
- identify ineffective recruitment strategies
- identify effective recruitment strategies

Learn from the experiences of others

These top tips of what to do and what not to do will guide you in developing a process for recruiting or can help improve what you are already doing. With more organizations sharing information and networking on issues related to the nursing shortage, it is easy to find out what others are doing that works or doesn't work. Once you identify processes, start developing your own list, and share it amongst the managers in your organization.

Top 10 things not to do in recruitment

1. Don't make statements about the work environment that are not true

We all want our workplaces to sound like the place to be, but exaggerating and misrepresenting what you have to offer is inappropriate. Attentive, newly hired nurses are going to realize very quickly that the picture you painted at the interview is not what they are seeing.

Therefore, be realistic and honest about your work setting: We all have employees who we wish worked for another department, and many of us hope for the day when we can update the physical layout or appearance of the workplace. Although you don't want to emphasize these points, respond honestly to the questions posed to you at interviews.

Case study: Be honest

Prospective employee: "How do people around here get along with each other? At the last place I worked, some nurses were hostile to one another."

Manager: "We realize the importance of a professional work environment and never tolerate hostile-type behavior in any of our departments. But, as you know, there will always be some people with behaviors that may make you uncomfortable. Part of my job, which I take very seriously, is to be responsive to staff when they identify unacceptable behaviors. I cannot recall any scenarios where we had hostility issues amongst our team here, but we have had our disagreements, as everyone does at times."

---

2. Don't make promises you cannot keep

Between completing interview sheets, giving tours of the facility, and answering benefit questions, it becomes quite a task to remember all that transpires during the interview process, including what was said. However, the nurses you interview will not forget what you tell them with regard to their schedule, wages, benefits, and so on. If you tell an interviewee, who informs you that he or she has already bought plane tickets, that if they are hired you can grant his or her request for Christmas off, you have trapped yourself and the rest of your staff. Therefore, always think the situation through, and imagine various "what if" scenarios. What if a staff member is out on medical leave and another delivers her baby two months early? How are you going to keep your promise for the new hire to still have the holiday off? How will staff with whom you currently work feel about a new hire getting Christmas off?

Instead of making verbal promises, put in writing anything you do promise, and mail or give the person you interviewed a copy of the document.

3. Don't allow recruitment to overshadow retention

Recruitment has long been the focus in nursing, particularly considering the state of the nursing shortage. But increasingly lavish incentives thrown at new nurses can rankle existing employees and make them feel abandoned and ignored. Don't offer incentives and attention to new employees at the expense of those you already have.

Pay attention to your advertising in newspapers and other venues, as not only job seekers will see these ads—your current staff will as well. Therefore, include your retention efforts in those advertisements. Also incorporate an internal advertising campaign to promote retention. Creating a workplace culture that focuses on retention is one of your best recruitment strategies.

4. Don't allow staff with unacceptable behavior to continue "bad mouthing" the department or organization

Set very clear expectations with all staff regarding this behavior, as it not only damages staff morale but also diminishes recruitment and retention efforts. Always remember, if they are willing to express negative opinions about the organization at work, just imagine what they are saying in the checkout line at the grocery store. A good place to start working on this issue is with staff who are in a charge- or supervisor-type position. Work with them through role playing and scripting for appropriate responses that will help to squelch this unacceptable behavior. Encourage staff to address negative comments on the spot, and direct individuals making the complaints to a forum where their complaints can be addressed, such as at staff meetings.

5. Don't use a 'licensed warm body' as a criterion for meeting recruitment goals

Numerous pressures are placed on recruiters and hiring managers to meet recruitment quotas and goals. Some units may feel so desperate that they resort to saying, "If they're licensed and breathing, hire them." It's tempting to interview and hire anyone who meets the minimum criteria, particularly for high-demand positions, but don't fall into that trap. The long-term costs in turnover, team morale, and productivity can be extreme if you hire an individual who doesn't fit. Most employees will tell you they would rather work short-staffed than bring the wrong team member on board.

One strategy to consider is to use temporary staff until you find the right professional for your unit. Reassure recruiters, managers, and staff that although it is important to get the position filled, it is critical that you fill it with a person who can contribute significantly to your organizational goal of quality patient care.

6. Don't dwell on your or your organization's limitations

Some organizations seem to have all the bells and whistles when it comes to recruiting, and the grass often looks greener in a competing facility, but be sure to focus on your organization's strengths. What keeps you there? Ask new and seasoned staff the same question. Talk these points up with potential candidates. Identify organizational limitations, and develop strategies for improvement.

7. Don't neglect recruitment infrastructure

It's amazing how many people think recruiters live glamorous lives, and how exciting it must be to travel and talk with people. But in reality, there are many functions and responsibilities included in the role and it can be lonely and challenging, especially if you're the only one in your organization doing it.

Set a long-term goal to develop a recruitment army. Equip employees in your organization to share the benefits of working there, and work with your staff development department to design a "My Stories" seminar. Encourage each employee in your organization to participate and to develop personal stories about how they make a difference in your organization. Discuss forums where these could be shared in public, such as cookouts, community gatherings, and letters to the editor of your local newspaper. Hold a follow-up group session to discuss responses.

Establish a community healthcare roundtable group to discuss healthcare personnel recruitment issues. Conduct regional work force analysis to identify high-priority personnel needs. If you know nursing will be a long-term need, work with nursing programs to increase enrollment and graduations. Work together to develop creative work force development programs, and apply collectively for funding from the U.S. Department of Labor, the U.S. Health Resources and Services Administration, or even private philanthropies that focus on healthcare access.

8. Don't expect sign-on incentives to retain staff

Sign-on bonuses can get an active or passive job seeker's attention, but most likely they will not be the sole reason an individual will agree to work with you. They can help motivate new hires to stay for the length of the sign-on agreement, but you must have a great work culture to retain them long term.

9. Don't allow units to operate revolving recruitment doors

Maintain turnover data on a unit basis. Identify units that have high turnover rates and determine what's causing the turnover. Analyze employee satisfaction and exit interview data, and compare and contrast findings among the different units. Meet with the unit manager and employees to discuss the data, and identify issues that might influence employee retention. Develop an action plan. Identify a responsible and accountable employee or committee to develop a timeline and oversee its implementation.

10. Don't spend time on strategies that aren't producing recruits

Analyze your recruitment strategies to determine which are producing results and which are not. You can add codes to the advertisements you place in a variety of media so you can determine how candidates learned about your openings. When potential candidates contact your recruitment office, ask them to describe where they saw the advertisement or provide you with the advertisement code. When you exhibit at career fairs, get an estimate of the number of people who attend the fair, the number who stop by your booth, the number who leave names and addresses, and the number who actually interview with you. If strategies are not producing desired results, consider setting them aside. Of course, one of your aims is to promote a positive image and create good will, so not all strategies will produce concrete results. But your time is valuable, and you want to make sure your total efforts produce recruitment results.

Top 10 things to do in recruitment

1. Do improve your interviewing skills

How you present yourself and the questions you pose during the interview process affect the perceptions of the prospective hire. Be prepared for the interview by having your desk presentable, having important documents on hand (such as the job description), and ensuring uninterrupted time, when possible. Seek input from the staff regarding questions they would like to see included during the interview. Don't discount the idea of also having staff members interview the candidate—after all, they are the ones who will be working side by side with the new nurse. The interview process should not be one-sided, so provide candidates with time to conduct their own interviews of you and the department.

2. Do involve staff in all recruitment processes

Giving staff the opportunity to be involved in the interview process is just one method of getting them involved in recruitment. Ask staff to preview advertisements before they go to print to offer a reality check, and make sure you are not promoting a process that doesn't actually take place in the department. Encourage staff members to accompany the recruiter to recruitment fairs or to meet with high school seniors on career day.

Make time to educate staff members on the correct response to the questions that are most commonly posed to the recruiter. Your staff will be unable to do their part in recruitment if they are not well-versed on matters such as employee benefits and new community services. Share with them what types of social situations are great opportunities for recruitment, such as when they hear about a new coworker at a family member's job whose spouse "happens to be a nurse."

3. Do identify and know your competition

Conduct a competition analysis to identify organizations you compete with for different types of personnel. Compare and contrast work cultures, opportunities for advancement, and types of units, specialties, and programs. Know the strengths of your organization, and be enthusiastic about sharing information on your outstanding programs and retention rates. Never make negative statements or comments about your competition; instead, redirect the conversation to discuss more positive aspects of your organization.

4. Do optimize Internet and e-recruitment technologies

Organizations are recruiting large proportions of healthcare professionals through use of the Internet. Make sure your "job opportunities" button is on your organization's home page and that it links directly to up-do-date, user-friendly job listings. Allow for immediate submission of applications and resumes online, and offer to answer questions by e-mail or by phone. Most hospital and healthcare Web sites are designed to attract patients, so review your site to make sure it also provides positive images that attract potential candidates. Stay away from spam recruitment messages, but certainly consider low-cost e-cards as an alternative to direct-mail campaigns. Look for strategies to keep you informed on the latest electronic recruiting technologies and, for major initiatives, consider outsourcing to high-tech recruitment agencies.

5. Do publicly brag about your outstanding staff in newspaper articles, journals, and other venues

Job-hunting nurses want to know about staff with whom they may work. When they read about staff who have attained certifications or volunteered for a community effort, they receive a message that the organization supports nursing. The more they see these public declarations of accomplishments, the stronger their perception that your organization supports its nurses and offers many opportunities. It also directly affects retention, as staff members love the accolades they receive when people they know see a photo or advertisement in the paper about their new certification. When announcing major physical changes to the organization, include photos of staff members, along with pictures of the upgraded facility.

6. Do embrace opportunities to work with schools of nursing

Due to the shortage of faculty at schools of nursing, many are having trouble meeting their classroom goals, as well as those for the clinical setting. Collaborate with the school of nursing, and create a wonderful opportunity to showcase student nurses all you have to offer in your facility. During their clinical rotations, students will be working alongside your nurses and will be able to picture themselves there as a staff member. During their time on duty, existing staff members will be able to get a feel for the characters and personalities of the prospective hires. Should they decide to apply for a position with you when they graduate, you will already have an idea whether you want them as part of the team. Remember, skills can often be taught later on, but character and passion for nursing must be there from the beginning.

7. Do set a personal goal to develop every inquiry into a job application

When you make the first contact with a prospective hire—whether a face-to-face meeting at a career fair exhibit or an e-mail or phone inquiry—set a personal goal that this individual will visit your office for an interview. Of course, he or she must meet the job requirements for the position, but with recruiting experience and expertise, you often can determine within the first moments whether the candidate is a good fit for your organization. Keep your own tally of how many got away and how many were hired.

8. Do market your organization in a thousand places rather than one

It's wise to remember the old saying, "Don't put your eggs in one basket," when considering marketing your organization. That is, don't invest your entire advertising budget in one resource, such as a newspaper or journal. Rather, use several media outlets to increase your individual and target group reach. Use a variety of media and face-to-face strategies to get the word out about how great it is to work with your organization. Consider marketing strategies such as trumpeting your Magnet designation or any national unit and specialty recognition awards. These types of outside recognition validate quality care and excellent workplaces.

9. Do establish trusting relationships

Honesty and integrity are two of the most important qualities of a great recruiter. Relationships with recruits begin at your first point of contact. Although it may be difficult to do so on a day-to-day basis, make sure you are attentive and fully engaged in the moment. Listen to their interests and concerns. Keep hiring managers informed of prospects, and provide consistent follow-up. Be professional and collegial with peer recruiters. If a prospect's background and skills are a better fit for a competing organization in your region, make the referral by giving your peer recruiter a call. Think about it: The prospect was not a good fit for your organization, but if they are a good fit for the other facility, you suddenly have two individuals at your competitor's organization singing your organization's praises.

10. Do spend time with colleagues who mentor, coach, and suggest ways to improve your recruitment skills

Everyone must seek ways to improve, and mentors are a wonderful way to fast track your learning and development. Identify areas you would like to improve, and then consider leaders who can help develop this expertise, which may come in the form of knowledge or it may be professional contacts. Be aware that the mentors who may help you most may be outside of your normal practice arena. Spend time with people who build you up, rather than tear you down.

Chapter 13

WHAT'S WORKING IN THE NONHEALTHCARE ENVIRONMENT?

Learning objectives

After reading this chapter, the participant should be able to

- identify recruitment and retention methods that have proven successful outside the healthcare environment
- compare basic recruitment and retention principles from the general workplace to those from nursing

Differentiate yourself from your competitors

Healthcare is a world of rules, regulations, and requirements specific to our service. We tend to stay within our own group when looking for resources, answers, and ideas on how to improve what we do. Managers participate in seminars geared only for the world of healthcare, and the journals they read are directed at the same audience. Sometimes we forget there is another world out there dealing with the same management challenges we have, including recruitment and retention.

For example, it is not easy to recruit and retain people to work at a fast-food restaurant chain when there are six more companies just like them on the same street. These companies address the same questions of how to compete when everyone pays the same starting wage.

Or they put money and time into orienting new people, just as in healthcare, only to find employees lured away to a place that will pay them more. Other industries also face the challenge of meeting difficult scheduling needs. For example, would you want to be working by yourself at a convenience store on the midnight shift and have to close out the cash register? We have more in common with other industries than most of us realize, and it's time to look at how the other side of the business world confronts some of these challenges successfully.

Surprising the customer

Many leadership lessons can be learned from observing what nonhealthcare organizations do to encourage their employees, and many of these successful principles could be applied to healthcare.

Case study: Checking in

I was checking in at the front desk of a hotel, when suddenly the young woman who was helping me stepped out from behind the counter. I thought she was heading that way to do something else, and I was taken aback when I realized she was simply coming around to talk to me. She handed me my room key and discussed local information. When I inquired about why she stepped from behind the counter, she shared with me that her company's goal is to make the customer feel special and like an individual, and they realized that talking to the customer from behind a desk is very impersonal. I was very impressed by this attitude, but I wondered how the employees felt about doing it. The young woman replied that she thought it was a great idea, as she had never liked having a counter between her and the people she was helping. The hotel kept me as a customer, even though they charged more per night then many others.

Customer service

You can see parallels between this behavior and those in your own workplace. Imagine if one of your employees approached the receptionist in personnel with a question about her paycheck. The receptionist is on the phone when the nurse approaches, and it is obvious that she is on a personal call. How important would you feel to the organization if you were this nurse taking time from your break to do this? Compare that to the receptionist who concludes the call quickly and makes immediate eye contact with that nurse. It sends a message that the employee is important and has your attention right now.

Case study: Shared goals

I arrived at a supply store a few minutes before they were due to open. It was a nice day, so I decided to wait outside for the short period of time. Looking into the front window, I noticed that all the employees gathered around one person for what looked like a meeting. When it was over, just before they unlocked the doors, I noticed all the staff got together and applauded. After completing my shopping, I asked the man at the check out about what I had witnessed through the windows. He informed me that it was their daily "pep" talk with their manager and that the applause was them congratulating one another for meeting a team goal that they had set.

Teams are made up of individuals

Making staff feel part of a team is a crucial element for retention, but if no one recognizes what people bring to the table as individuals, where is the motivation to hang around with the organization? At change of shift in your department, make time to recognize what the group and individuals have accomplished. The team leader or charge nurse can do so in your absence, not necessarily every day, but on a regular basis to encourage and motivate staff.

Keeping up with the changing workplace

"This isn't your grandfather's workplace. We're five years into the new millennium and businesses everywhere are changing with the times." —Amanda C. Kooser[1]

One of nursing's greatest challenges continues to be its difficulty in changing with the times and moving past old habits of management. Keeping up with the changing work force is essential to successful businesses and has allowed them not only to attract the best employees, but to keep them around as well. Concepts that appeal to the changing work force include telecommuting, job sharing, and flexible work hours and days.

Value employees as people

In this day and age of computers, we find ourselves moving away from pen and paper. Although e-mail communication is effective, sometimes a handwritten note can accomplish much more: It sends a message that you took the extra time to hand write a message of importance.

An electronic instrument manufacturer started a "You Done Good Award," which is simply a printed note card that employees can send to one another. The cards have become important enough to the organization and people who work there that those who receive one display it proudly on their desk. The communications manager for this company noted that even when people say nice things to you, it means more when people take the time to write their name on a piece of paper to say it.[2]

Recognition

In some car-producing companies, employees involved in the manufacturing process get to actually sign their name on some part of the product. It is a representation of their involvement in developing this product.

For example, you can walk onto a Southwest Airlines aircraft and see a plaque in the cabin recognizing an employee for loyalty of service. In each monthly issue of the airline's magazine, there is a story with a photo about one of the employees and how he or she has contributed to the success of the company. Whether it is autographing a product or putting the employee's photo in a magazine, the recognition is clear to everyone, especially that employee.

Spirit of fun

Some industries have discovered the value of making the workplace fun. Southwest Airlines' employees work hard, but they have fun at the same time. The company encourages committees that arrange fun employee activities, and although they are in a very serious business, staff know that acceptable humor at the right time is supported and encouraged from the top.

Other examples of ways employers have incorporated fun into the workplace include the following:

- A small, privately owned manufacturing company produces products that require extreme concentration at the individual workstations. Unannounced, the manager showed up with several rented vans and shut down the shop for part of the day. He took everyone out for ice cream and then to an arcade, where he handed each person tokens to play the games.

- A group of government employees had been working hard toward meeting a team goal that they eventually achieved. One afternoon, they were called into the manager's office and handed movie tickets for that afternoon's show. The spontaneous act made the employees feel like kids playing hooky from school and allowed them to have fun as a group.[3]

- A kitchen appliance assembly plant is located in the stifling South of the country. Despite the presence of fans, during the summer, it is a challenge for the employees to stay motivated and meet production expectations. One day, employees see one of the managers walking through the plant handing out popsicles—simple yet important to the staff.

These examples may seem impossible to duplicate in healthcare—you can't shut down a medical-surgical floor to take people to a bowling alley. But it's important to note that it is not so much what you do as how unexpected the action is.

When you read the business section of the newspaper, start looking for stories about what other businesses are doing to recognize, recruit, and retain employees. Although you may not be able to do exactly the same things they are doing, their actions should help you come up with some great ideas of your own. How about initiating an employee support account for each department's budget that gives the manager funds throughout the year to purchase items such as movie tickets, ice cream, pizza deliveries, or pens? Surprise the staff with the unexpected, and the return on your investment will show up in your retention statistics.

Use your Web site

A quick Internet search of many well-known corporations with reputations for success in the area of recruitment and retention reveals one important fact: The companies have pages on their Web sites dedicated to the individual and team achievements of their employees. Some have employee photos, quotes, information on the charities the employees select to sponsor, photos of company events, and so on.

Many health organizations have Web sites, and it is time to take advantage of the power of the Internet. Use this opportunity to show employees that they are so integral to the operation of the hospital that you are posting employee photos, accomplishments, and achievements right on the Web site. People love to go online or call their families and friends to tell them to look on the hospital Web site for their picture or story.

Best places to work

Business magazines publish lists each year of the "best places to work" in America. The magazines use specific criteria such as benefits, wages, and work flexibility in the selection process. *Fortune* magazine announced its 2005 winner, Wegmans, a grocery store chain based in Rochester, NY, and stated, "Wegmans does things differently, including the way it deals with employees."[4]

The Wegmans Web site offers 16 good reasons to work there, which range from friendly teams to adoption assistance. "In order to attract and retain the best people, we offer competitive benefits that make the perfect garnish to the employment experience."[5]

Pizza Hut was voted the best place to work in Dallas by Dallas/Ft Worth Magazine, and the company proudly proclaims, "The only thing that tops our pizza is our people!" The company believes in providing an environment that nurtures staff and makes them feel that they have contributed to the process. The eight leadership principles followed by the company include encouraging everyone to contribute their ideas and state, "We hate bureaucracy and all the nonsense that comes with it."[6]

Auto rental company Avis uses the motto, "We try harder." Of its employees, 18,000 enjoyed the opportunity to be entered into a program that recognized the top 40 examples of who had tried harder. Prizes were awarded and their stories posted on the Web site.

How the employee perceives they are being treated and how you actually treat them may be worlds apart, and it is vital that organizations explore this difference. "If you want the customer to be treated like a king, then you have to treat the people you manage like royalty."[7] In Bill Fromm's book, *The 10 Commandments of Business and How to Break Them*, he reflects on a client he had who was rude to his employees to the point of using profanities. Some employees hated coming to work if they knew they were going to have to deal with this client. As the well-being of his people was Fromm's biggest priority, he "fired" the client. Fromm gathered his employees at a meeting, where he announced that he had terminated the relationship with the client. He was received with screams of surprise and applause by his employees, who felt supported by their boss.

Once again, it may seem impossible to relate these examples to your workplace, but with patience and input from the staff, you will be amazed at the difference you can make. Managers need to step up and support and protect those who do their job every day.

Case study: Sometimes the customer isn't right

I had an experience in one of my management positions where a patient who was scheduled for an outpatient procedure in surgery was so rude that she reduced one of the night nurses to tears. Nothing staff could do for her was right in her eyes, and who would put an unhappy customer to sleep with anesthesia in this day and age of liability? The surgeon agreed that the risk was not worth taking, so he canceled the procedure and the patient was discharged home. You should have seen the look on the employees' faces and the disbelief that someone stuck up for them. I hope I never have to "fire" another patient, but doing the right thing for employees sometimes takes precedence, even in healthcare. How else will employees know that they actually matter to the organization if management isn't there to support them?

Strategies to make new employees feel welcome

Have you ever considered how much it costs your organization in time and money to orient one nurse? Many businesses have put a price on orientation and initial training and have related these costs to a sum that equals what they put into recruitment and retention efforts. Would doing anything less make good business sense? Once you have them and they want the job, how important do you make them feel once they are on board? How would you like to start your first day as a new manager with not even a pad of paper on the desk? Remember, you need to put the same efforts for recruitment and retention into the new manager you hire as you do for the staff-level nurse.

We can learn techniques from the business world to improve our welcome to new nurse managers:

• Have business cards made and ready to go on the first day

• Have the office stocked with office supplies, such as pens, a stapler, and paper

- Place on the desk an updated company directory of phone numbers and e-mail addresses, their pager/cell phone with instructions and numbers, and a welcome note from the organization with a jar of candy

- Arrange for another manager to show up at lunch time to take the new employee to lunch

- Be sure the computer is in working order and that personal information from the previous manager is removed

- Arrange a manager's breakfast or lunch meeting to introduce the new manager to his or her peer group

- If new managers relocate from another part of the country, mail them packets of information about the community from the Chamber of Commerce, provide them with contact information for reliable realtors, and inquire as to whether they need information about the local schools, places of worship, and other community information

Other techniques employed by businesses to make a good first impression include the following:

- Intel Corporation sends its new hires a packet of material in the mail before they begin employment that reads "Welcome to the World of Intel."

- Gift baskets are sent to the homes of new hires for Quick Solutions.

- An e-mail is sent to all employees of Persistence Software informing them that today a new employee is starting. The company encourages existing staff to stop by to introduce themselves by placing a tray of breakfast food near the new hire's desk.[8]

All the ideas and creativity you read about should lead you to this one thought: Your ability to show employees that you care about them is an important advantage when faced with the challenges of holding on to good staff and recruiting the best out there looking for jobs.

Regardless of what it costs you in time and money, the effectiveness and success of your actions will be in the emotion of the employees. If they feel like you care about them being a part of your team, you have made an emotional connection with people and will find that they are committed members of the organization.

References

1. Amanda C. Kooser, "Workplace 2005," *Entrepreneur,* February 2005.

2. Bob Nelson, *1001 Ways to Reward Employees* (New York: Workman Publishing, 1994): 4.

3. Beverly Kaye, et al., *Love 'Em or Lose 'Em* (San Francisco: Berrett-Koehler Publishers, 1999): 90.

4. Matthew Boyle, "The Wegman Way," *Fortune, www.fortune.com/fortune/bestcompanies* (accessed August 2, 2005).

5. Wegmans Web site *www.wegmans.com/about/jobs/benefits.asp* (accessed August 2, 2005).

6. Pizza Hut Web site *www.pizzahut.com/about/careers/* (accessed August 2, 2005).

7. Bill Fromm, *The 10 Commandments of Business and How to Break Them* (New York: Berkley Books, 1991).

8. Leigh Branham, *Keeping the People Who Keep You In Business* (New York: AMACOM, 2001).

Additional resources and reference tools

Timothy Butler, et al., "Job Sculpting: The Art of Retaining Your Best People," *Harvard Business Review* (September–October 1999).

Robert E. Farrell, *Give 'Em the Pickle,* Portland: Farrel's Pickle Production, Inc., 1995.

Adrian Gostick, et al., *Managing With Carrots,* Salt Lake City: Gibbs-Smith Publisher, 2001.

Bob Nelson, *1001 Ways to Energize Employees,* New York: Workman Publishing, 1994.

Web resources

www.humanresources.about.com	Extensive resource for all matters related to managing
www.shiftwork.com	Resources for staff who work night shift
www.followyourdreams.com	Daily motivational statements, quotes
www.hru.net	Monthly manager tip
www.managementfirst.com	HR articles, tips, etc.
www.growtalent.com	Survey results on best places to work
www.fastcompany.com	Resource for innovative business practices

NURSING EDUCATION INSTRUCTIONAL GUIDE

Target audience

Nurse Managers
VPs of Nursing
Chief Nursing Officers
Directors of Nursing
Nursing Home Administrators
HR Directors
Nurse Recruiters

Statement of need

This book provides an educational study guide that will help nurse managers recruit and retain staff. The nursing shortage is a huge problem and facilities are offering high salaries and signing bonuses simply to get nurses in the door. This book provides strategies not only to recruit nurses but to also retain them once they are through the door. It describes strategies to encourage professional development, support managers and employees, develop reward and recognition programs, and ways to create an employee- and family-friendly environment.

Educational objectives

Upon completion of this activity, participants should be able to do the following:

- Identify the major disadvantages of high staff turnover
- Identify characteristics of a diverse work force
- Discuss strategies for managing diversity in your organization
- Identify strategies to support and develop nurse managers
- Recognize warning signs that a new nurse manager is in need of support, guidance, and direction
- Implement strategies managers can use to show staff that you make time for them
- Discuss strategies that promote an employee-friendly workplace
- Discuss program examples that leave a perception with staff that their employer is family-friendly
- Identify the components of professional models of care
- Discuss the benefits of professional models of care
- Identify ways to implement quality workplace improvement systems
- Evaluate the results of implementing quality workplace improvement systems
- Identify effective methods of promoting collaborative practice between nursing, medicine, and other professional departments
- Discuss the benefits when nursing staff actively participate in collaborative systems and processes related to patient care
- Identify education and training resources related to professional development
- Discuss how a commitment to professional development aids recruitment and retention
- Identify ways to reward staff for exceptional performance
- List essential aspects of the performance review that enhance retention
- Identify methods to recruit young people into healthcare careers
- Discuss the value of establishing relationships with schools of nursing
- Identify the value of using metrics to measure recruitment and retention success
- List examples of recruitment and retention data that are useful to manage your work force
- Identify ineffective recruitment strategies

- Identify effective recruitment strategies
- Identify recruitment and retention methods that have proven successful outside the healthcare environment
- Compare basic recruitment and retention principles from the general workplace to those from nursing

Authors

Shelley Cohen, RN, BS, CEN, and Dennis Sherrod, EdD, RN

Accreditation/designation statement

This educational activity for three contact hours is provided by HCPro, Inc. HCPro is accredited as a provider of continuing nursing education by the American Nurses Credentialing Center's Commission on Accreditation.

Disclosure statements

Shelley Cohen and Dennis Sherrod have declared that they have no commercial/financial vested interest in this activity.

Instructions

In order to be eligible to receive your nursing contact hour(s) for this activity, you are required to do the following:

1. Read the book
2. Complete the exam
3. Complete the evaluation
4. Provide your contact information in the space provided on the exam and evaluation
5. Submit the exam and evaluation to HCPro, Inc.

Please provide all of the information requested above and mail or fax your completed exam, program evaluation, and contact information to

> Robin L. Flynn
> Manager, Continuing Education
> HCPro, Inc.
> 200 Hoods Lane
> P.O. Box 1168
> Marblehead, MA 01945
> Fax: 781/639-0179

If you have any questions, please contact Robin Flynn at 781/639-1872 or *rflynn@hcpro.com.*

Nursing education exam

Name: _____

Title: _____

Facility name: _____

Address: _____

Address: _____

City: _____ State: _____ ZIP: _____

Phone number: _____ Fax number: _____

E-mail: _____

Nursing license number: _____

(ANCC requires a unique identifier for each learner)

1. Which of these options is not a benefit of reducing a facility's turnover?

   a. Cost savings due to reduced need for expensive orientation and training of new nurses

   b. Reduced stress on other staff members

   c. Increased time for managers to spend supporting existing employees

   d. Increased patient census

2. Diversity characteristics combine to form

   a. unique identities for each of your staff

   b. additional challenges for the unit manager

   c. similar response patterns, as the majority of nurses are female

   d. group polarity and conflict

3. The most effective strategy for incorporating diverse staff into your unit is

   a. conformity

   b. superficial assimilation

   c. mutual adaptation

   d. ethnocentrism

4. It is vital for administration to support the middle manager through

   a. ongoing leadership development

   b. scheduled time to meet with his or her manager

   c. clear expectations

   d. all of the above

5. Which of the following is not a warning sign that a nurse manager needs more direction?

  a. Staff members often approach other managers with their problems

  b. The manager frequently cancels meetings with his or her supervisor

  c. The manager has difficulty focusing on tasks

  d. The manager misses one deadline

6. One strategy to show staff a manager makes time for them on a constant basis is

  a. an annual performance review

  b. being available at the change of shift

  c. sending an e-mail

  d. staff meetings

7. One of the most important strategies for promoting an employee-friendly workplace is to

  a. know staff and colleague life priorities and motivators

  b. allow for personality flaws and negative staff interactions

  c. begin staff meetings with "what's wrong with this unit" stories

  d. tell them they have bad breath

8. Which of the following is not a family-friendly benefit or program?

  a. Pet health insurance

  b. Adoption assistance

  c. Mandatory overtime

  d. Phased retirement

9. A professional model of care that can aid retention is

  a. split bureaucracy

  b. shared governance

  c. diversified leadership

  d. shift bidding

10. Which of the following is not a benefit of professional models of care?

  a. Quality care

  b. Safe care

c. Nurse retention

d. Higher turnover rates

11. A primary focus for implementing workplace improvement is to

a. teach teams to work together

b. determine employee desires

c. improve numerous systems and processes concurrently

d. base workplace improvements on data and information

12. The data collection method that focuses on organizational or unit strengths and capabilities to achieve improvement goals is known as

a. appreciative inquiry

b. performance appraisal

c. incremental interview

d. employee satisfaction survey

13. A synonym for collaborative is

a. mutual

b. same

c. one way

d. independent

14. The active involvement of nursing in processes related to patient care results in

a. more complaining from the staff

b. longer length of time to resolve problems

c. improved retention of nursing

d. less accountability from staff

15. Which of the following is not an effective resource for the staff nurse looking to enhance his or her professional development?

a. Continuing education

b. Attending inservice meetings without actively participating

c. Participating in professional organizations

d. Role models

16. **Recruitment and retention efforts are aided when the organization**

   a. requires the nurse to pay 100% of continuing education costs

   b. provides no scheduling flexibility to attend professional development programs

   c. offers ongoing support for continuing education on-site

   d. expects the nurse to independently seek resources to enhance his or her professionalism

17. **The best rewards for exceptional performance are**

   a. expected

   b. expensive

   c. genuine

   d. simple

18. **Performance reviews can enhance retention when**

   a. nothing negative is discussed

   b. both the manager and employee are prepared for the review

   c. the manager does not use goal setting

   d. the employee is not required to change any behaviors

19. **The reason most often cited by youth for choosing nursing careers is**

   a. the opportunity to work in a number of geographical locations

   b. nurses are autonomous decision-makers

   c. helping people or making a difference in their lives

   d. the variety of work settings

20. **Schools of nursing are integral to recruitment because they provide**

   a. a renewable resource for nurse professionals

   b. an opportunity for staff nurses to serve as preceptors

   c. free student nurse labor on units

   d. faculty consultants

21. **Metrics are important to recruitment and retention success because they**

   a. measure turnover

   b. provide endless numerical possibilities

   c. serve as key indicators for strategic decision-making

   d. define average length of service

22. An example of a recruitment metric is

a. turnover rate

b. position requisitions received and filled

c. years of experience

d. length of orientation

23. An example of an ineffective recruitment strategy is to

a. under promise and over deliver

b. embellish organizational benefits

c. develop recruitment infrastructure

d. delete recruitment strategies that are not producing results

24. An example of an effective recruitment strategy is to

a. involve staff in the recruitment process

b. use little or no Internet and electronic technologies

c. advertise only in your local newspaper

d. remember that it is impolite to brag about your organization

25. Successful recruitment and retention strategies used in the non-healthcare work environment include

a. non-flexible benefit packages

b. rules that prevent employees from sharing cultural celebrations

c. maintaining a serious work environment at all times

d. making employees feel a part of a team

26. An important workplace principle that healthcare can benefit from embracing is

a. to treat the people you manage like royalty

b. to recognize the customer is always right and that the employee needs to accept that

c. that new managers should not be pampered or catered to in their first few days of work

d. that you should never allow yourself to have employees with an emotional connection to their employer

Nursing education evaluation

Name: _____

Title: _____

Facility name: _____

Address: _____

Address: _____

City: _____ State: _____ ZIP: ____

Phone number: _____ Fax number: _____

E-mail: _____

Nursing license number: _____
(ANCC requires a unique identifier for each learner)

I. This activity met the following learning objectives:

Identified the major disadvantages of high staff turnover
Strongly disagree   1   2   3   4   5   Strongly agree

Identified characteristics of a diverse work force
Strongly disagree   1   2   3   4   5   Strongly agree

Discussed strategies for managing diversity in your organization
Strongly disagree   1   2   3   4   5   Strongly agree

Identified strategies to support and develop nurse managers
Strongly disagree   1   2   3   4   5   Strongly agree

Recognize warning signs that a new nurse manager is in need of support, guidance, and direction
Strongly disagree   1   2   3   4   5   Strongly agree

Implemented strategies managers can use to show staff that you make time for them
Strongly disagree   1   2   3   4   5   Strongly agree

Discussed strategies that promote an employee-friendly workplace
Strongly disagree   1   2   3   4   5   Strongly agree

Discussed program examples that leave a perception with staff that their employer is family-friendly
Strongly disagree   1   2   3   4   5   Strongly agree

Identified the components of professional models of care
Strongly disagree   1   2   3   4   5   Strongly agree

Discussed the benefits of professional models of care
Strongly disagree   1   2   3   4   5   Strongly agree

Identified ways to implement quality workplace improvement systems
Strongly disagree   1   2   3   4   5   Strongly agree

Evaluated the results of implementing quality workplace improvement systems
Strongly disagree   1   2   3   4   5   Strongly agree

Identified effective methods of promoting collaborative practice between nursing, medicine, and other professional departments
Strongly disagree   1   2   3   4   5   Strongly agree

Discussed the benefits when nursing staff actively participate in collaborative systems and processes related to patient care
Strongly disagree   1   2   3   4   5   Strongly agree

Identified education and training resources related to professional development
Strongly disagree   1   2   3   4   5   Strongly agree

Discussed how a commitment to professional development aids recruitment and retention
Strongly disagree   1   2   3   4   5   Strongly agree

Identified ways to reward staff for exceptional performance
Strongly disagree   1   2   3   4   5   Strongly agree

Listed essential aspects of the performance review that enhance retention
Strongly disagree   1   2   3   4   5   Strongly agree

Identified methods to recruit young people into healthcare careers
Strongly disagree   1   2   3   4   5   Strongly agree

Discussed the value of establishing relationships with schools of nursing
Strongly disagree   1   2   3   4   5   Strongly agree

Identified the value of using metrics to measure recruitment and retention success
Strongly disagree   1   2   3   4   5   Strongly agree

Listed examples of recruitment and retention data that are useful to manage your workforce
Strongly disagree   1   2   3   4   5   Strongly agree

Identified ineffective recruitment strategies
Strongly disagree   1   2   3   4   5   Strongly agree

Identified effective recruitment strategies
Strongly disagree   1   2   3   4   5   Strongly agree

Identified recruitment and retention methods that have proven successful outside the healthcare environment
Strongly disagree   1   2   3   4   5   Strongly agree

Compared basic recruitment and retention principles from the general workplace to those from nursing
Strongly disagree   1   2   3   4   5   Strongly agree

2. Objectives were related to the overall purpose/goal of the activity

Strongly disagree   1   2   3   4   5   Strongly agree

3. This activity was related to my nursing activity needs

Strongly disagree   1   2   3   4   5   Strongly agree

4. The exam for the activity was an accurate test of the knowledge gained

Strongly disagree   1   2   3   4   5   Strongly agree

5. The activity avoided commercial bias or influence

Strongly disagree   1   2   3   4   5   Strongly agree

6. This activity met my expectations

Strongly disagree   1   2   3   4   5   Strongly agree

7. Will this learning activity enhance your professional nursing practice?

Yes

No

8. This educational method was an appropriate delivery tool for the nursing/clinical audience

Strongly disagree   I   2   3   4   5   Strongly agree

9. How committed are you to making the behavioral changes suggested in this activity?

a) Very committed

b) Somewhat committed

c) Not committed

10. Please provide us with your degree

a) ADN

b) BSN

c) MSN

d) Other, please state:

11. Please provide us with your credentials

a) LVN

b) LPN

c) RN

d) NP

e) Other, please state:

12. The fact that this product provides nursing contact hours influenced my decision to buy it

Strongly disagree   I   2   3   4   5   Strongly agree

13. I found the process of obtaining my continuing education credits for this activity easy to complete

Strongly disagree   I   2   3   4   5   Strongly agree

14. If you did not find the process easy to complete, which of the following areas did you find the most difficult?

a) Understanding the content of the activity

b) Understanding the instructions

c) Completing the exam

d) Completing the evaluation

e) Other, please state:

15. How much time did it take for you to complete this activity (including reading the book and completing the exam and the evaluation)? _____

16. If you have any comments on this activity, process, or selection of topics for nursing CE, please note them below.

17. Would you be interested in participating as a pilot tester for the development of future HCPro nursing education activities?

Yes

No

Thank you for completing this evaluation of our nursing CE activity.